As For Tomorrow, I Cannot Say

As For Tomorrow, I Cannot Say

Thirty-three years with multiple sclerosis

Diana Neutze

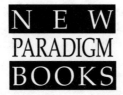

In loving memory of Paul

ISBN 1-877270-17-2
ISBN 1-892138-06-9

Published in the United States of America by
NEW PARADIGM BOOKS
22783 South State Road 7, Suite 97, Boca Raton, FL 33428
Tel.: (561) 482-5971
FAX: (561) 852-8322
E-mail: jdc@flinet.com
Website: http://www.newpara.com

Published in New Zealand by Hazard Press Limited
P.O. Box 2151, Christchurch, New Zealand
email: quentin@hazard.co.nz
www.hazard.co.nz

Contents

Chapter 1

August, 1966. Guy and I, with our four-year-old son, Paul, went to northern France to study cathedrals: Rouen, Amiens, Rheims, Laon, Paris, Chartres. That sounds memorable enough. And certainly, it has left me with stunning memories: standing at the crossing of Amiens cathedral unable to see the ceiling of the aisles so that it looked as if the whole building soared to the height of the nave, upwards and upwards, bathed in the morning light streaming down from the clerestory; or Paul's later revelation that he believed, if you went to church, you had to stay in a hotel. But the journey was memorable for quite other reasons.

While we were in France, Guy's struggle with an inherited obsessional disorder became so intrusive that he agreed to see a psychiatrist on our return to London, which led later to a three-month stay in a rehabilitation unit and a slow return to normal health. It would be true to say that, for him, the holiday constituted a beginning. For me, on the other hand, it was an ending. The Buddhists have the image of a gateless gate, a gate you pass through without realising that there is a gate at all. The world on the far side, however, has changed completely. The light falls differently. Our holiday in France was, for me, a gateless gate. I left London believing I was a healthy woman and returned a week later, although I didn't then know it, with the first symptoms of a chronic, degenerative illness. I would never be the same again.

My symptoms came on gradually and, initially, were all to do with the sensory nerves. At first, I experienced an irritation of the hands. I thought that I needed a hand cream. And when, back in London, I went to a doctor, he assumed I had an allergy and gave me anti-histamine. The next symptom was that I was crossing the garden of La Musée des Beaux-Arts in Rouen, when it felt as if my stomach muscles had disappeared. Notice the 'as if': neurological symptoms are very difficult to describe. What really happened, probably, was that I experienced a cold feeling: my ability to distinguish hot and cold had been impaired.

We returned to London and several weeks passed; although I didn't actually feel ill, I did feel uneasy and insecure. Then we were given an elderly piano by friends who were going back to New Zealand. I had played the piano since I was eight, although in the seven years since I was married I had had to content myself with playing whenever I visited a friend who happened to have an instrument. But now at last, I had one of my own. On Sunday afternoon, I threw everyone out – we had a cousin and his wife staying – and I sat down to play. I started with the works I had played at a friend's only a few weeks before: Bach's Italian Concerto and the first movement of Beethoven's Pathétique sonata. It didn't take me long to realise that I had reached a stage where I needed more practice. Resignedly, but still contented, I had a go at an easier Mozart sonata. But I couldn't play that either. Feeling increasingly anxious, I tried a C major scale. But it was no good; even that was beyond me. I sat at the piano in cold desperation. The afternoon, which I had expected to be so enjoyable, settled bleakly around me.

I went to the doctor the very next day.

'I can't use my hands,' I said in great distress.

He neither examined me nor asked me any questions. All he told me was that I was a very nice woman, that I had a very nice husband and a very nice son. He told me to go home and read *The Art of Positive Thinking*, and he wrote me out a prescription for tranquillisers. I had been labelled an hysteric. Some weeks before our French cathedral holiday, Guy had developed a very stiff neck, for which the same doctor had given him arthritis pills. But the stiff neck had nothing to do with arthritis. Guy had an obsessive fear of brain damage: he had come to be afraid that walking would jar his brain, rattle it about in his brain box. So he had taken to walking very gingerly to protect his brain and this had given him a stiff neck. Although Guy was suffering from a neurosis, the doctor assumed, because he was a man, that he had a physical problem. I had a serious physical problem but I was a woman and, therefore, neurotic.

I came home from the doctor's feeling worse than ever. Inevitably, when I told Guy and my cousins what the doctor had said, they believed him. I was obviously neurotic and, therefore, they kept an eye on me, humoured me but did not encourage me to talk about how I felt because that would be dwelling on things. Thus began a month or so of nightmare. I didn't read *The Art of Positive Thinking* but I did swallow the tranquillisers. I'd wake each morning feeling jangled and reach for the pill bottle. I now realise that the noise of the alarm clock was affecting me: sensory nerve damage had turned me into a tuning fork.

I was to experience a similar negative reaction to Mahler symphonies. Guy had just discovered Mahler and wanted to share his enthusiasm but I wasn't a taker. I was accused of being reactionary and lacking in musical adventurousness. One evening when I was on my own – the cousins had by now moved out – I thought I'd make a determined effort so set myself to listen to Mahler's 5th. But it defeated me; it set my teeth on edge and I just didn't like it. High violins against equally high woodwind did nothing for my sensory nerves but, as I didn't know that, I was a self-declared philistine.

Sensory nerve damage wasn't all I was enduring. Fine-tuning in my hands was also a problem. I did not feel at all confident that I could hold on to Paul adequately when we were about to leave a London bus; I kept depositing already dropped bus tickets; I picked up three plates, as I thought, but in reality, took only two and left the third on the table; washing Paul's jeans by hand, I found it well nigh impossible to wring them out. I foolishly filled a hot water bottle without resting the base on the table and it fell out of my insecure grip. (Luckily, it fell outward or I would have added severe burns to my other problems.)

About this time, our landlord insisted we paint the flat. One morning I climbed up onto the table with my pot of paint in my hand, intending to tackle the elaborate mantelpiece surround. However, I overbalanced and fell off. As if the mess of spilled paint was not enough, I became almost hysterical, which only confirmed everyone's belief in my neuroticism. The shuddering jar of my fall had really distressed me, set me totally on edge. I was given the afternoon off and went to Primrose Hill where I sat looking out over the city, filled with shame and utter bewilderment. I just didn't understand what was happening to me.

From time to time, I tried to get Guy to acknowledge the changes in my life. I'd show him my handwriting, for instance. 'Look at this,' I'd say, 'it's positively geriatric.' And he'd nod understandingly, without understanding at all.

I might have gone on like this indefinitely, struggling against a malaise that became more all-encompassing with every week. But one Sunday at the laundrette, I bent to pick up a clothes basket of wet, but spun, washing, and my stomach muscles revolted; they simply refused to respond. With great reluctance, I went back to the unconcerned doctor.

'I just don't feel well,' I volunteered, with none of the previous visit's distress in my voice.

This time, although he still didn't ask any questions, he did examine my eyes. Without saying anything, he wrote out a referral to the Maida Vale Hospital for Nervous Diseases. I didn't have to wait very long for an appointment. It all seemed routine, until Dr Marshall, the neurologist, held up a finger.

'Touch my finger and then touch your nose,' he instructed me.

I reached out towards him and watched in disbelief as my right hand wavered hopelessly off target. I could touch my own nose but no matter how hard I tried, I couldn't touch his finger. My co-ordination was completely shot.

Dr Marshall didn't say anything but sent me off to get dressed again. I must have taken too long because he came to investigate the reason for the delay. He very gently did up my top blouse buttons, over which I had been struggling to no avail. We returned to his office, I still aghast at my co-ordination failure.

'I want you to come into the hospital for further examination,' he informed me.

In a daze, I agreed and by the end of the next week, I entered the hospital. Guy was very distressed and indeed when we got to the admission lobby, the nurse assumed he was to be the patient.

I was instructed to get undressed and into bed and told I was to be given, almost immediately, a lumbar puncture. I'd heard about them and knew they were unpleasant but before I had time to really panic, a young woman came across from the other side of the room to reassure me that, although the procedure was upsetting, it didn't last all that long. Certainly, it was physically most unpleasant, a horrid feeling of pressure, but probably no nastier than having one's sinuses washed out. But there was also the mental recoil because my spine was being invaded, a sort of instinctive fastidiousness. It is essential, after a lumbar puncture, to remain lying down for 24 hours and to drink a great deal to replace the fluid removed from the spine. Otherwise, one can experience a very severe headache.

Apart from when Paul was born, I had never been in hospital. As most neurological illnesses are chronic, not to say degenerative, the mood of a neurological ward is heavy with fear and hopelessness. I didn't then know what was the matter with me and I fully expected to get well, so all my compassion was directed outwards to my fellow patients and their predicament. I was haunted by Othello's cry: 'But yet the pity of it, Iago!'

Following my lumbar puncture, I was prescribed steroids, a daily injection of ACTH, on a diminishing dose. Steroids, as I was told, don't make you better, but if you are going to get better, they make you recover more quickly. They also make you hyperactive, so I required sleeping pills if I was going to get any rest at all.

In the end, I stayed only a week in the hospital. Dr Marshall wanted me to stay longer.

'What can you do for me that can't be done at home?' I wanted to know.

'We can look after you,' he said.

But Paul had given up eating while I was away and I insisted on going home. A district nurse was appointed to give me my daily steroid injection on alternate buttocks, with a remission of sins on Sunday. When there is a four-year-old watching a needle being jabbed into your bum each day, you can't grumble; you have to act as if this is a normal and pleasant experience. As well, a home help came in for two hours twice a week. Guy took Paul to nursery school on his way to work and friends or neighbours collected him and entertained him for a while so he wasn't left with a bed-ridden mother for too long before his father got home. He was very good and would sit up in bed beside me to watch *Blue Peter* or *Animal Magic* on television.

All the practical aspects were set in place. It was now up to me to get better. But it was a long haul. Whether my sight was affected or not, I don't know – it hasn't been since – but I couldn't read. The tuning fork effect meant I didn't want to listen to music or watch TV. I had nothing to do but lie there. Our London flat consisted of a kitchen, a bathroom and two large rooms, one of which was Paul's; the other was our bed-sitting room. The divan, which was our bed, faced into the room. I don't know why I didn't ask to have it moved, even at the cost of changing the whole room round, so I could look out the window at the wonderful trees. Some days, I asked Guy to prop up a painting where I could study it, but mostly I just lay there from 10 a.m. till 4 p.m. Apart from Alice, our upstairs neighbour, I had scarcely any visitors but had to endure all on my own.

And it was endurance. I suppose the steroids had kicked in because I jangled. All day the nerves ran, a current from one nerve length to another. I used to say that if you could have attached a battery to me, with all that electricity, the housework would have been done in no time. Then I developed what is called l'Hermitte's sign: whenever I bent my head on to my chest, I experienced a graunching, like a particularly bad gear change, down my spine. And if this wasn't enough, I sweated profusely. I changed my night clothes several times a day because I was wringing wet. I started wearing Guy's pyjamas, as I'd run out of my own nightwear.

Lying there all alone with nothing to do except jangle and sweat, I developed the tendency, if a plane went over, to tense up in expectation that a bomb was about to fall. I had been a child in New Zealand during the Second World War but now I was experiencing my own inner blitz.

There were many days when I'd ring Alice before I went to the lavatory and ask her, if I hadn't rung back within 10 minutes, to come down and check up on me. One day, following a visit by ambulance to Dr Marshall, I felt as if I were suspended by a hook from the ceiling and slowly rotating – decidedly unsafe. One of my friends was doing research for her PhD, so I rang and asked her to work from my place that day. She read and took notes at our kitchen table, while I 'rotated'.

My Sunday break from the steroid became increasingly difficult. I suppose it would be true to say that I had withdrawal symptoms. I must have been an enormous burden on Paul and Guy, but they managed gallantly. Paul and I devised extraordinary methods for doing such things as tying his shoelaces. I tried to be as helpful as possible, patiently carrying things out to the kitchen one at a time, because of my unreliable hands, and organising from the bed, but I was, of necessity, very dependent. I don't remember taking baths but I do know that, because of the gear changes up and down my spine, I couldn't wash my hair. Ours was a 19th-century London house, so it had no shower; hair washing had to be done in the handbasin.

I'd organise my own lunch. Once or twice I decided on a scrambled or poached egg. This meant breaking the egg into the bowl with one hand. I'd seen it done often enough on TV but I could not do it. There would be the broken egg and there would be quantities of shell and it would take me the next five minutes to fish these out of the bowl. After this had happened a couple of times, I decided against eggs for lunch.

When my cousin's wife visited one day she brought with her a friend, who studied me for a bit then asked: 'You are going to get better?'

The complete certainty of my positive answer haunts me now.

The weeks went past and I started, slowly, to recover. As the function of my hands returned, I asked the West Indian nurse what I could do to hasten their recovery.

'Wring out your smalls,' she advised me.

I didn't fancy that, but I borrowed some of Paul's plasticene and I'd sit of an evening watching TV, which, by now, I could do without too much distress, rolling the plasticene around in my fingers.

I reached the stage where I felt up to getting dressed, instead of spending all day in bed. The look of joy on Paul's face, when he came home from nursery school and saw me back to normal, was very telling. It had obviously been harder for him than we had realised. I had been so occupied with my endurance and my slow recovery, and Guy with all the added responsibility, that we had not given enough thought as to how my illness must be affecting a four-year-old.

But at last, I was better, or rather I had completed my course of injections, and the home help was no longer deemed necessary, I no longer jangled and sweated my way through every day. I was weak and fragile, I still needed the sleeping pills – it was to take a while before I could wean myself off my dependence on them – but I was able to resume my normal life: looking after my family and teaching part time.

First there was Christmas, a brief mid-winter holiday. I wanted to get Guy a Delacroix print, which meant a visit to the National Gallery in Trafalgar Square. I had felt overwhelmed the first few times I had ventured out after the weeks in bed, but that was only the short distance to collect Paul from nursery school. To get the print, I had to brave a bus and all the London pre-Christmas crowds. I was determined, however, and I did manage it even though, on the bus on the way home, my fingers curled so tightly round the strap of my shoulder bag that I couldn't disengage them.

And Christmas food buying was an ordeal. That year, we spent a couple of days with New Zealand friends, but there was still a lot of shopping for the three of us. I was coming down the hill with my loaded trolley and I must have looked very fragile as a neighbour came to my rescue and took the trolley from me. She wasn't even someone I knew well, although I did get to know her better later on. I don't even know how she knew I'd been ill, although Jack, our cockney milkman, was very concerned. He took to bringing the milk in each day and putting it in the fridge instead of leaving it at the door, so perhaps he had told my neighbour.

Before I started back at my part-time teaching job, I had another hospital check-up. I admitted that, while I had recovered physically, only needing now to build up my strength – there was hardly a day when Guy didn't monitor my co-ordination by holding up his finger for me and greet with relief my ability to touch it competently – I was feeling far from my usual self. When I saw acquaintances ahead of me while I was out shopping, I was crossing the street to avoid having to talk to them. It was not surprising, after all I had had to contend with, that I was suffering from post-reactive depression. Dr Marshall prescribed anti-depressants. My first reaction to them was alarming: when I walked, it felt as if the pavement was coming up to meet me. It seemed so like a neurological symptom that I became really anxious. I took a day off teaching, an unpolitic reaction that alarmed the organiser of the coaching institute – crammer to the English – where I taught into thinking I was going to be as unreliable as in the previous term. I rang Dr Marshall, who persuaded me to persevere and the unpleasant symptom did disappear after a couple of days. I took the anti-depressants for a few months but I don't like taking medication and I weaned myself off them as soon as I could, swallowing two out of three tablets a day, then reducing the dose to only one tablet, then nothing. Certainly, I was free of the tablets well before the hospital expected.

In all this time, I hadn't asked what had been the matter with me. But, now, as I was almost completely recovered, I did.

'Have I got disseminated sclerosis?' (This was how multiple sclerosis was described back then.)

'There are lots of forms of sclerosis, just as there are lots of forms of cancer,' I was told.

I was so taken aback that I didn't tell Dr Marshall not to prevaricate. I don't know whether he chose to side-step my question because of the rather patronising attitudes manifested towards patients in those days or because he had gathered from me that Guy was at a crisis point in the struggle with his obsessions and thought, therefore, that I had enough to contend with. But although he didn't tell me the truth, he did explain that I'd had a virus in the spine, which might recur, and if it did, I might not recover. As I was in remission, I ignored the subjunctive and let myself be lulled into believing that the illness would never recur. I have since read of various so-called cures of the initial phases of multiple sclerosis, including hyperbaric oxygen, but it would appear that if you have the exacerbating/remitting kind of illness, not knowing and carrying on as normal also has the desired result. In other words, it wouldn't really matter what you did.

Chapter 2

By now, we were well into 1967. I carried on with my life as normal, teaching part-time at the crammer and studying for a Post-graduate Certificate of Education by correspondence. I was recovered but Guy, after looking after me so assiduously, could no longer cope. His condition deteriorated dramatically, and in October, a full year after my hospitalisation, he was admitted for three months to Roffey Park, a rehabilitation unit in Sussex.

I continued in remission. Guy continued to check my co-ordination. In our ignorance, we believed that, if the virus struck again, it would strike in exactly the same way. We didn't then understand that the nervous system is extensive and that it's not always the same area that is affected.

After Guy's crisis I started meditating. I had been lurching between spells of anxiety/tension and spells of being in the dumps and recognised I needed to do something about this. I was, as always, unwilling to take medication. Because of the Beatles, meditation was very much in the news so I decided I would give it a go for a year and then decide whether it was doing me any good. Other people I knew took it up but dropped it after a few weeks, but I practised assiduously twice a day for a year, by which time I was completely hooked. My afternoon practice was during Paul's – now aged six – television programmes, so he was happily occupied. He became very efficient at telling telephone callers: 'Mummy's meditating. Can she call you back?' I have meditated for 20 of the more than 30 years that have passed since then.

The meditation people recommended a very basic form of yoga as a way of preliminary relaxation, so I started my afternoon practice with quarter of an hour of very unproficient yoga. In 1969, however, we returned to New Zealand, Paul and I for three months and Guy for one, and when we got back to London, I decided to attend a small Iyengar yoga class. One lesson was enough. I knew this was for me. I started practising at home immediately and, even now, when I am so disabled, I practise physical yoga for at least an hour a day. Although I didn't then, I now realise why I was so instantly won over: yoga is about stretching and my body recognised how much I needed to stretch. Just at the time that I started yoga, I acquired a job at a comprehensive school in Margaret Drabble's 'ever-weeping Paddington'. Before I could begin, I had to have a medical. The powers-that-be, it seemed, had never heard of a virus in the spine. I was weighed and measured. For the measurement, I had to stand against the wall and a lever was lowered onto my head.

'Five foot four and a bit.'

'But I'm five foot five and a half,' I protested.

'See for yourself.'

He was right. It seemed that despite my age, only 30, my spine had shrunk. I didn't at the time associate this with the illness, but some two years later, when I was about to be employed to teach yoga at an evening class, I had to submit to another medical. Same room, different medical officer. I stood to be measured. Five foot five and a half. The years of yoga had uncompacted my spine and stretched me back to my correct height.

I started yoga in February and in July, Iyengar himself came to London for a month's intensive teaching. I duly went to a beginners' class and some guardian angel prompted me to speak to him afterwards.

'I have a virus in the spine,' I volunteered timidly.

'I'm not a doctor,' he snapped. 'I have to see you work.'

Intimidated, I stammered that I had been in that afternoon's class. He directed me to talk to one of his London teachers. I went home and thought no more about it. But when I went to my usual Friday class, my tutor Penny said in great relief, 'Thank goodness you've come. He's been asking for you.'

It appeared I was to attend the next afternoon's class, considerably more advanced. The lesson started with a head stand, which I was excused, as I hadn't at that stage ventured to do this. The shoulder stand that followed, however, lasted 20-30 minutes, twice what I was used to. But if that was demanding, it was nothing compared with what was to come: the standing poses. There are some eight of these and I was really put through my paces. For each pose, Iyengar, who called me Virus, worked me, on the first side, to the limit. Then, for the second side, he'd be checking out other people. I would try to gauge by the direction of his voice which way he was facing. I didn't know him then. He had the alertness and quickness of a wild animal. His energy levels were so potent that it seemed as if a wild panther was in the room. 'Virus,' he'd bellow and I knew that my slackening attention had been spotted and I'd try even harder.

After the standing poses, we sat to do twists. Suddenly he looked at me and barked, 'You've had enough. Go home!' From then on, I trusted him implicitly. If it was your mind that was blocking your doing a pose, he was fierce. But if it was your body, he was gentle. Two years after this episode, he said to me, 'I used to have to be gentle with you. Now I can shout.' Obviously, my stamina had improved considerably.

It was only a matter of weeks after his 1969 summer visit that the teachers' training class was set up, under the control of Iyengar's first lieutenant, Silva Mehta. A demand had arisen in London for yoga classes at the evening institutes of the Greater London Council. The man in charge, who had seen Iyengar demonstrate yoga poses, insisted on Iyengar-trained teachers but there were only about six for the whole of London. He contacted Iyengar, who, not entirely willingly, set up the training course that met for two to three hours twice a week. Although, by then, I had been learning for only six months, I went to the inaugural meeting. Because of the class where I'd been called Virus and put through the hoops, I had quite a high profile with the selection committee. As well, we were asked to come forward and teach a pose. I was given *Ardha Chandrasana*, half-moon pose. Because I have a verbal memory all I had to do was slot my mind into Penny's instruction and I could repeat what she said, word perfect. This impressed the selectors no end and I started the training course.

It was about this time that Guy, watching me practise my yoga, said he thought he could do it. I suggested he try and it wasn't long before he, too, was coming to the training class. With all this yoga, we felt less and less inclined to eat meat and we became vegetarians, although it took us a while to give up the weekend breakfast of bacon and eggs.

Our vegetarian diet, not one concentrating on milk, eggs and cheese, was immensely healthy; we avoided junk food and, instead, ate lots of fruit and vegetables. We ate brown rice, brown flour, wholemeal bread and pasta, brown sugar or honey. I stopped having low blood sugar. Previously, when I felt the usual faintness and disturbance of vision, I'd have to eat something immediately and I took to carrying glucose tablets about with me, wherever I went. After the reform of my diet, this glucose was replaced by nuts or cheese. I also found yoga helpful.

I'd get home from a day's teaching and feel the familiar symptoms coming on. But if I did an hour's yoga practice straight away, I was okay, even though it would take me, at the very least, another half-hour before we could eat. Without the yoga and without eating, I would have become more and more discombobulated.

You may well wonder what yoga and diet have to do with multiple sclerosis, but all the physical activity kept me, if not necessarily fit, immensely supple. It taught me to listen to, and trust, my body. I respected it, thought of it as an instrument, not a sexual object; it removed any coyness, invaluable now, when I have to be lifted on and off the lavatory.

There was a stage, after the MS had come out of remission, when I kept wanting to do a particular pose, one where you lie on your back, bend your knee, hook two fingers round your big toe, straighten your leg and then swing it over to the side as far as you can, without actually touching the floor.

'Why do I keep wanting to do this?' I asked the physio.

'Because it's the opposite of foetal spasticity,' she replied.

I have already mentioned that yoga helped to stretch me back to my proper height. Some years ago, when I was still standing, I asked a friend to measure me: five foot four and a half. She stayed during my yoga practice, so I asked her to measure me again when I was lying on the floor, when I could stretch myself out properly: five foot five. Out of curiosity, I bothered her once more after I had done my version of a shoulder stand, otherwise called half-plough with a chair: back to my proper height, five foot five and a half.

Years of practice have ensured that I have yoga hips, knees and ankles, very useful to prevent injury when I have fallen, often in a reef knot, or when, now, I am being moved and I end up in rather an ungainly position. I also have a yoga back, especially now when half my practice consists of a forward bend when I am lying along my legs. I once asked a younger friend if he could touch his toes. 'Yes,' he said, 'but with my hands, not my head.'

It would be true to say that yoga and a vegetarian diet kept me healthy. It is always a good idea not to draw the body's energies away from battling MS. Many of my deteriorations have been connected to other illnesses such as a duodenal ulcer or bladder infections brought about by catheterisation when I have been travelling. I know, as well, that my whole inner self has benefited from my doing yoga. I am a calmer, less stressed and anxious person. I can truly say that I don't know who I would be if I hadn't been meditating and doing yoga all these years. By learning to listen to my body's wisdom, I have come to feel that my body is my 'mostly companion'. Far from thinking that my body has let me down, I am convinced that it is fighting my multiple sclerosis for all it is worth.

So, in the first six years after the onset of my unnamed illness, we stayed in London and for the last three I was very involved with yoga. My health was so good that we tended to forget the ominous words that the illness might recur. Guy had stopped checking out my co-ordination.

Then in 1972, we returned permanently to New Zealand. Looking back, I can see all sorts of reasons why we should have stayed in London, but there we were back in Christchurch, somewhat alienated after 10 years away, with no money, no jobs, nowhere to live. We found an unfinished house on an undeveloped section on the Cashmere hills – unlined concrete block, two rooms and a bathroom (with no window), battered by the prevailing easterly but with a fabulous view; our friends christened it 'the garage', because it had started life as a double garage/basement but hadn't got any further. We had to have a moat to persuade rainwater to go round the house, instead of through it, on its way down the hill. We both taught yoga and I did some relieving teaching. We were appallingly broke, I was underachieving and, because of the smallness of our living quarters, we had no privacy. It was a great strain on my health and on our marriage. The marriage broke first. We separated in January 1976. By then I had started my PhD and was a teaching fellow at Canterbury University. This meant a more secure income, although it was still precarious.

Chapter 3

It was at the beginning of 1977 that I noticed a return of the nerve running. My co-ordination was still okay, but I was concerned enough to consult a doctor. I remember her glee at discovering that my ability to distinguish hot from cold was impaired. I lay on her consulting table while she splotted my stomach with hot and cold test tubes. I consistently guessed wrongly.

The doctor sent me to a neurologist, but, unfortunately, she chose an old-fashioned specimen who didn't believe in communicating with his patients. He had a posse of medical students with him. The consultation consisted mainly of questions, although I was asked to hold my arms out in front of me and the tremor in my hands was duly noted. However, as my father had the same tremor without any neurological complications, I failed to see the significance in that. The consultation was over. I had felt very frustrated at the specialist's failure to communicate with me and when I considered the other patients in the waiting room, none of whom looked confident enough to complain, I knew none of them would take the initiative. So I rang his receptionist to register my protest. I don't suppose she passed my grumble on, but I felt better having made the effort.

I went back to the doctor and she read me the neurologist's report: 'This patient has multiple sclerosis but, so far, is manifesting no hard neurological signs'. I blacked out in a state of shock. The doctor claimed that she thought I knew. When the news had broken about cellist Jacqueline du Pré having MS, I had wondered: her symptoms sounded uncomfortably like mine. Instead of being convinced that I had MS, however, I wrote to her recommending Iyengar yoga. Obviously, I believed that I owed my continuing good health to yoga. I suggested that she talk to fellow musician, Yehudi Menuhin, who claimed Iyengar had cured his bursitis. I received a standard secretarial reply, thanking me, along with thousands of others, for my interest.

Now, I was the one with MS. Guessing you may have an illness is very different from knowing you actually do have it. I could paraphrase

Dylan Thomas: ' it was my thirty-seventh year to heaven . . . and the weather turned round'.

I rang my brother-in-law, John, who was a doctor in Auckland. It became apparent from our conversation that he had suspected all along that I had MS. Then I remembered Dr Marshall telling me he had heard from my brother-in-law: one of the house surgeons in the Maida Vale hospital was from New Zealand and a friend of John's. He was the one who had reported that I was ill and what was the matter with me. John was appalled at the type of neurologist I had encountered; he stated categorically that I needed to consult one who would answer questions. But when I went back to my doctor requesting a second opinion, she was outraged.

'I'm not having patients who shop around,' she insisted.

I changed doctors. Friends recommended one whose style, I found, was completely different.

'I find MS a threatening illness,' he admitted. 'You'll expect me to make you well and I can't.'

I wasn't so stupid. My parents had a friend with MS and I knew it was chronic and degenerative, but not much else. The doctor gave me a neurological textbook.

'Come back,' he said, 'when you have questions.'

I learnt that MS was not a killer; I learnt about the myelin sheath that surrounds the nerves, like the plastic coating on an electric cord; I learnt of the two kinds of MS: the progressive, creeping paralysis type and the exacerbating/remitting type; I learnt that the severity of the first attack was a pointer towards later prognosis. And all the time, I was in shock. The first words that came into my conscious mind when I woke every morning were 'multiple sclerosis'. All my courage drained out of me. Instead of being in remission, it was as if I was already at some final, debilitating stage of the illness. Like a wounded insect, I dragged myself through the days: teaching, researching, looking after Paul, and doing yoga. I told only a few close friends and my obsession with my illness must have taxed their tolerance sadly.

Little by little, I recovered and my fighting spirit reappeared. My mother, who had osteo-arthritis, lay about on a sofa all day like a Victorian heroine. I used to wonder when the sal volatile was going to appear. I became determined that I wasn't going to be like her and adopt illness as a career. I had no vocation for it.

From feeling that I mustn't take any risks, must batten down all the hatches and scarcely venture a step out of doors, I came to recognise that I must, in fact, be adventurous, must do more rather than less. I must live as fully as possible while I was still able to. I didn't want to look back in later years and say 'if only I hadn't held myself back'. I wanted to feel my options were still open.

I was told I had MS in March. Sometime in May or June there was a Women's Convention in Christchurch, which I attended. At one plenary session I found myself voting against the majority. I felt the position the (unelected) committee was advising women to adopt was unethical and so I abstained. I refrained from raising my hand in favour while, all around me, women were enthusiastically endorsing the committee's attitude. I received many askance looks. I admit it would have been much harder to maintain my steadfastness if I'd had to raise my hand, while everyone else kept theirs lowered. I don't remember ever feeling so exhausted.

'You've had your Nuremberg experience,' a friend sympathised.

Two or three days later I paid the price. I had my second MS attack or exacerbation. I was cold and numb from the waist down. I told the doctor I felt as if I was prematurely decaying. And this time, my balance was much more affected; I felt all the time as if I was walking on a slippery surface. The doctor immediately put me on steroids: prednisone. This time it was pills instead of an injection but the effect was just as unpleasant: they hyped me up so much that I needed a tranquilliser to enable me to sleep.

This time, though, there was no question of my going into hospital. I asked the doctor what I could/should do.

'Carry on as normal,' he advised, 'but in case it's a virus, don't overdo it.'

So, with a great fear in my heart, I carried on. This time I knew what was wrong with me and that I might never recover totally. However, I went about my daily life. I tutored, researched, sang in a choir, taught and did yoga, took the dog for a walk on the hills, looked after Paul, who, by this time, was nearly 15. It must have been appalling for him, bearing the brunt on his own. He needed support himself and yet he was the one giving it. One night when there'd been a particularly gruelling choir practice – we'd been made to stand a lot and we'd run over time – in the car, on the way home, I broke into noisy, jerky sobs;

no gentle trickling of tears, but the whole McCoy. I parked the car and felt I'd calmed down enough to go into the house; I didn't want Paul to be distressed by my distress. But I had overestimated my control. I no sooner got inside than I started weeping again. Instead of retreating in panic, Paul came and knelt beside me. He held me until the sobbing ceased and I was calm enough to go to bed.

If that was how one member of my family responded, it was quite different when I told my mother about my illness. Certainly, she cried out in pain, but otherwise it was as if she was wondering why this had to happen to her. I knew she lived vicariously through me, but this was ridiculous. As one of my friends said, I was refusing to be ill and in a wheelchair, so everyone could be sorry for my mother.

At length, my brother took issue with her. 'What are you doing for Diana in all this?' he asked.

She tried to make amends. She offered to sell the big family house and move into something smaller and more compact, which could subsequently be adapted for me. I refused her offer. It was not yet necessary to live as if I were disabled.

Obviously, the fact that I was decidedly off colour didn't register with most people. I had, after all, told only my closest friends that I had MS. I don't know whether the secrecy helped or not, but I rather think it did. I wasn't visibly disabled and I didn't have to deal with what felt like prurient curiosity. But it was heartbreakingly difficult. The only bright spot was the fact that, this time, my hands weren't affected and I could still play the piano. The walk with the dog on the hills, previously a joy, now became an ordeal because of my impaired balance.

Yoga was particularly difficult. Iyengar used to say, 'Do this, this and this; then the lightness comes.' For me, it was all heaviness. There is one pose I particularly remember struggling with day after day. In *Jatara Parivatasana* you lie on your back with your arms stretched out as if you are being crucified. On an out breath, you raise your legs to 90 degrees, then on another out breath, you lower them towards your right hand, holding them steady about an inch above it. In order to stop your whole body collapsing to the right, you have to work your stomach muscles to the left. At the same time, you lean heavily on your left elbow. It is a pose that is very good for the digestive system and the lower back. When I was well, it was a pose I especially liked; it took so much control and bodily awareness to get it right. But at the stage of my second attack, the pose became indescribably nasty to do. There was no longer pleasure to be derived from the feeling of control. When your body from the waist down is cold and numb, every movement of the stomach muscles is a torture.

Then, one day when I reluctantly prepared, as in the previous four to six weeks, to do this pose, something had changed. Instead of the expected heaviness, the lightness had returned and I could once more revel in my body's control. All the symptoms had rolled off and I was completely recovered. It doesn't make sense that it was just at this moment that I registered I was better, but that is how it was. Despite the dread I had been living with that, this time, there would be residual damage, I had for a second time gone into remission.

For the next weeks, I lived in what I can only call a state of grace: the reprieve from permanent illness and disability was so miraculous. Everything I did, I did with full awareness. And I am not just talking about lovely things like playing the piano or taking the dog for a walk on the hills; the feeling was just as intense for mundane tasks like doing the dishes or taking the rubbish bags out. It was a profoundly religious experience, a time of epiphany. I think this is how we're supposed to live, focused and there. So, now, when things are going badly with me, I don't read or listen to music. I stay quietly, focused on the present moment. The past may be unpleasant, the future scary, but now I am looking out my window at the light streaming through my walnut tree, I'm watching the birds at the feeder. Now is perfectly okay.

> if this day were to be my last I would die
> loving
> the long shadows of autumn
> as light filters through the apricot tree –
> celebrating
> the chattering flight of a fantail –
> rejoicing
> in the architectural splendour
> of a Bach partita
> arch after musical arch soaring upwards

The state of grace lasted some four weeks; it eventually came to an end when I developed flu. Its aura, though, is still with me. I have retained a hunger for a way of life when I was able to get out of my own way. I now know what is possible. Thus began eight extraordinary years. I was once more in remission but, this time, I knew what I was in remission from. I couldn't take anything for granted: playing the piano, walking on the beach, dancing were all special. They might one day be taken from me, but for now I could do them and rejoice in that doing. As one of my friends put it, I lived with an edge.

Chapter 4

I completed my PhD in 1978 and, after giving a paper at a conference in Brisbane, applied for a position as tutor at Melbourne University. I was accepted and made arrangements to go there the following year. Paul decided that he wasn't ready for Australia and opted to stay in New Zealand. He was loath to leave Christchurch, but finally agreed to go and live with his father in Wellington.

I knew no one in Melbourne, although various people gave me names of their friends I could look up. With my second MS attack only 18 months behind me, I knew I was taking a risk. And this would be the first time I'd ever lived on my own. Still, true to my recognition that I needed to live more fully, to push out my limitations, I went ahead. After all, if it didn't work out, I would just have to come home with my tail between my legs.

One thing did bother me: so far, I had told only my closest friends that I had MS. If I went to Melbourne and made a number of new friends, I felt I must tell them right from the start and not just dump it on them after a number of months, or when I had yet another exacerbation. 'Oh, by the way, did you know I happen to have MS?' They needed to choose if they wanted to know me. But, because I'd had no experience in telling acquaintances, I decided I'd practise. I had been invited to a farewell tea by a fellow PhD student, whom I didn't know very well. So, halfway through the evening, I thought the time was right.

'I have multiple sclerosis,' I told her.

I spoke portentously, as if Chopin's Funeral March was playing in the background. She just looked at me. There was no change in her expression and she didn't say a word. I don't know to this day whether she was ignorant about MS and didn't like to ask or whether she was embarrassed and wished I'd shut up. Finding her silence very unnerving I wittered on, giving her a great deal of information she'd no doubt rather not have had.

When I got home and was cleaning my teeth, I looked at myself in the mirror. 'You didn't get that right,' I told myself.

The next night I was invited to another farewell tea. This time I dropped the fact of my having MS into the conversation casually, mentioning it only in passing with no more emotion than if I'd been announcing I had ingrown toenails. But what I had forgotten was that my hostess played the cello, and knew of Jacqueline du Pré.

'Diana,' she said in absolute horror, 'you do know what it means?'

So, I'd got it wrong again. Portentousness didn't work, but neither did flippancy. And, after all, if my doctor found it a threatening illness, other people with even less knowledge were going to find it even harder to deal with. There was no right way to tell people; it depended partly on their level of receptivity. Mostly, however, I adopted a wry tone. People wanted neither high tragedy nor offhandedness, but they could cope with black humour. I've been told I shouldn't take responsibility for others and seek to protect them, but if I don't I may have to cope with their ineptitude. Protecting them may be easier than dealing with crassness or avoidance.

Anyway, I went to Melbourne and made lots of friends, especially among the students. I coped with telling people I had MS, and they coped with hearing I had it. One woman said I was dealing with it with 'dignity and grace'. I wasn't so sure about that, but I liked the phrase. Because I had been in remission for so long and because of the yoga and vegetarian diet, friends tended to believe it was something I was doing that kept me so well. Indeed, I began to think the same way myself. This mistaken belief was to give me a great deal of trouble later on when the MS began to rampage. In the meantime, though, I was well and the resulting *hubris* was of no account. Far from having to come home with my tail between my legs, my five years in Melbourne were splendid.

After a while, I became used to living on my own, although, at first, it was very difficult. I was lonely. Hardly a Saturday morning passed without my feeling thoroughly out of sorts. In the end, I decided to test myself. I'd walk to the Victoria Market. If I felt worse when I got home, then there really was something the matter with me: perhaps I was going down with flu. If I felt better, it was because I was suffering from a low-level depression and the walk, the colour and liveliness of the market had lifted my spirits. I always felt better.

Then again, I kept being haunted by the expectation that I should be having a different sort of life. On Fridays and Saturdays, for example, I'd feel convinced that everyone else was out having a whale of a time and that there was something wrong with me because I was stuck at home on my own. But then I examined what was happening. The rest of the week my evenings were very pleasantly spent reading and playing the piano. Why could I not enjoy Friday and Saturday the same way? If I removed the expectation that, somehow, on those evenings, I should be doing something different, maybe I'd find them all right too. It worked. I started enjoying Friday and Saturday evenings as much as any other.

I read an article about loneliness. It claimed there was a calibrated scale with extreme loneliness at one end and solitude at the other. Extreme loneliness was toxic and tended to drive people away. It was creativity that converted loneliness into solitude. I found it needn't be anything as significant as writing an epic; trying a new recipe or buying some petunia plants at the market and putting them in pots on the windowsill so the snails wouldn't get them was sufficiently creative to tip me into solitude.

My tutoring appointment was for three years. I was completely autonomous. I was told the year's syllabus and teaching timetable and left to get on with it. My work included seminars for second years and a little lecturing. I liked the teaching; I enjoyed the relaxed informality of Australian students; I had a most attractive flat in north Melbourne, within walking distance of the university; I had a delightful tortoiseshell tabby called Polly. In my second year there, Paul came over to Australia and went up to Mount Oak, a commune south-west of Canberra. There was a great deal of richness in my life. Eventually I was teaching yoga, had joined a choir that specialised in the music of Bach and was a member of the Jung Society. The MS existed for me only as a shadow. Only on really hot days, and Melbourne could certainly produce them, did I feel precarious, uncertain whether I was going to trip over my own toes or whether I could skibble across the road in time. But basically, I was very well and the shadow was no more than a storm cloud well down on the horizon.

The three years ended. Mischievously, I reapplied for my tutorship: if they reappointed me for another three years, they'd have to pay me more and give me tenure. A staff meeting passed a hasty resolution: no tutor could be reappointed. I was out of work but I stayed on in Melbourne for another two years, eking out the dole by occasional private teaching and teaching yoga.

Looking back over those two years, I can now see that I used them to slow myself down, to adopt a different attitude to time. I had to rethink, had to create, myself.

My days were spent with yoga and meditation, playing the piano and singing, both in a choir and duets with a friend, reading, doing a very beautiful tapestry that Paul had given me and walking in the park. In those days, I wasn't writing poetry but I did spend half an hour a day recording my dreams or writing up my journal. I became very actively involved with the Jung Society, having occasional sessions with a Jungian analyst and practising Jung's active imagination to good effect. When I had first started meditating in London, I had stirred up a lot of unfinished business from the past. The meditation experts were dismissive. 'It's possible to tip-toe through a herd of sleeping elephants without waking them,' I was told.

But I had woken them; they were rampaging. Now, when I started paying close attention to my dreams, more unfinished business from the past emerged. The analyst didn't want to deal with it himself but he recommended a programme, which I followed conscientiously. I took the phone off the hook. Then I sat at the typewriter for half an hour detailing some aspect of our life in London, round the time of the onset of my multiple sclerosis and Guy's time in the rehabilitation unit. Next, I played the piano for half an hour in whatever mood was appropriate, always anger or grief. Lastly, I danced for 30 minutes. This programme proved very effective. The day I wrote about the beginnings of the MS, I sobbed like a heart-broken child for the whole hour and a half. I was utterly exhausted.

At the end of several months, I had a dream. I came down the front steps of our London house and went to inspect the rubbish bins. All three had just been emptied and had sparkling clean, new bin liners; under the privet hedge lily of the valley was growing. I had cleared away all the detritus of the past, and my rubbish bins were all ready to receive more litter. I subsequently used the image in a poem: 'in my mind's untidy corner/ garbage accumulates/ and no lily of the valley grows'.

My changed perspective on time took a while to establish itself. After all, I had been used to being very busy and committed to my university work. I sat one day in the sun with a cup of camomile tea, intending to play the piano at 11 o'clock. Three minutes before the hour, Polly, my little cat, came and sat on my knee. Still a slave to time, I was about to put her off at 11 o'clock sharp, when I realised what I was doing. I laughed at myself and sat there with her purring contentedly for another 10 minutes, until she decided of her own accord to get down. I had only myself to please. I didn't have to meet any deadlines. I could make time serve me instead of my having to serve time.

The years in Melbourne had been very fulfilling, but it was time to return to Christchurch. My parents were ageing and, besides, I had been commissioned to write the centennial history of the University of Canterbury's School of Engineering. I came back, bringing with me Polly and my ancient VW.

Chapter 5

The money I earned from writing the engineering history was scant so, as well as teaching yoga, I went back to tutoring at the university. I found a flat not far from my parents' house. It had stairs but I was well, wasn't I, so that was all right. And, even if I was going to deteriorate some day in the future, I didn't want to live now as if I was already ill.

I settled happily into my new routine of researching and teaching but with various much-loved activities from the past, such as walking on the beach or along the tracks beside the Summit Road. Everything seemed to be going well until I started developing unexplained back pains. Now, it must be remembered that the woman with backache was one who practised an hour and a half of yoga a day and had done so for 15 years; she had also spent long hours on analysing her dreams and believed very strongly that illness was a product of the mind. I was fully convinced, therefore, that I could, and would, solve the problem of my back pain on my own. Many a night I'd get up after only a couple of hours' sleep, drink a cup of herb tea and write in my journal. The pain would ease and I'd go back to sleep, convinced, mistakenly as it turned out, that my journal writing had been the necessary trigger. Then, to compound my difficulties, my MS symptoms reappeared. Looking back, I don't think I was having a full-scale exacerbation, but that was what I believed at the time. I felt completely defeated. Yoga, meditation, vegetarianism, dream work and journal writing were not sufficient, it seemed. At some deep level, I was choosing to be ill. I worried endlessly about what possible benefit the illness could be giving me. It was bad enough being ill; I blamed myself as well.

I did go to the doctor and once more was given prednisone, with the usual side effects. The MS did retreat, but not completely – walking on the beach became insecure; I even tried an anti-spasm drug, baclofen, for a short while until my natural antipathy to medication made me desist – and the back pain intensified. I had by this time seen a neurologist who was convinced that my back pain had nothing to do with the MS. My doctor experimented with various medications. In the end, he tried me on slow-release arthritis pills. By then, a friend who was house sitting had insisted I come and stay with her. She thought I was just too fragile to be living on my own. I had been there only a couple of days when I had a day of constant pain. By evening, it became necessary to call an after hours doctor, who promptly admitted me to hospital. I would like to say I was taken into hospital in the middle of the night – it sounds suitably melodramatic – but, actually, it was round 9 o'clock.

At first they wouldn't give me anything for the pain until they'd checked out I didn't have peritonitis. And then it took several days before they came up with a diagnosis. In the meantime, I was ordered bed rest, the worst thing that could have been suggested, given my incipient spasticity. Immobility would make my muscles even more inclined to spasm. But I was in a gastro-enteritis ward, not a neurological one. In the end, I was given a gastroscopy and it was discovered I had a duodenal ulcer. My doctor was mortified that this hadn't occurred to him – back pains are quite common in such cases – and claimed he couldn't face the fact that I had two serious illnesses. He also stated, and maintained almost to the end, that my ulcer was caused through repressed anger. My immediate, fierce disclaimer convinced him he was right. Indeed, I was not only angry, I was outraged. If he'd said stress, I would have accepted it. But, by calling it anger, he was discounting all the inner work I had done to come to terms with the MS, all the grieving. One day in Melbourne, when I knew I was going to have to spend time alone with my grief, it was as if I was wandering on my own through an Antarctic waste: cold, barren, desolate.

> it's a nightmare trudge
> on the edge of endurance
> while the parasite of cold
> eats into their bones
> space and time have lost all meaning –
> day after day in a torrent of sameness
> cascades over them –
> no unfurling season marks
> by bud or falling leaf
> their passage across the snow

People often asked me whether I didn't wonder why this had to happen to me, but I can honestly say the thought hadn't occurred to me. After all, why shouldn't it happen to me? By glibly assuming that I was angry, my doctor, it seemed, was making me out to be petty. Inevitably, I became angry which, to him, proved the point. The impasse this created damaged what had been a good relationship.

But here I was with a duodenal ulcer and slowly deteriorating MS. In time, the ulcer mostly cleared up, although not completely; I remained on a maintenance dose of medication for nearly 10 years. The MS didn't clear up. At first, it was suggested that, after a suitable interval, I would go back into remission, but this was not to be. My balance was greatly affected, I had sensory discomfort from the armpits down and a greater degree of bladder retention. Walking was becoming more and more difficult and it wasn't long before I needed walking sticks if I was crossing any large space where I could not easily locate myself by means of visual cues. For all that, maybe I would have got better if disaster hadn't struck.

It was 1 September 1985 when Guy rang to tell me Paul was in hospital in Canberra with severe liver failure. As soon as he could organise a passport, Guy flew over to see what could be done. After seeing Paul, he rang me in tears. He brought him back to Auckland on 16 September and I flew up that same day to be with him. I have come to regard any illness involving the liver as truly malignant. Because of the breakdown of the liver, fluid accumulated in Paul's gut, and his kidneys were under severe strain; with all the water weight he was carrying, he looked as though he were pregnant with quintuplets. He was appallingly ill. Guy didn't want to leave him, so he slept on a La-z-boy in his room while I stayed with my brother-in-law John and his wife Bev. When I visited the hospital, I had to use a wheelchair, as the distance from the car to Paul's bed was too great.

And all the time, Paul was getting worse. They used diuretics to try to drain away his excess fluid, catheterised him and restricted his liquid intake. I suggested we make the amount he was allowed to drink into ice cubes so he'd have to work longer at each swallow. Once the hospital had ascertained the extent of the damage to his liver, they consulted the DSIR and the botanical gardens and came up with a list of possible foods that would have caused the problem. It included comfrey which, indeed, he had eaten. The members of the commune had been growing it in one of their glasshouses and Paul had eaten it enthusiastically when it came into season, the way you'd eat silver beet. (I have a recipe in a herb book for *comfrey au gratin.*) The trouble was that Paul had eaten young, tender leaves, which would have been richer in the offending alkaloids that had induced the massive haemorrhaging in his liver.

But finding out what was the matter and how it had been caused brought us no nearer to solving the problem. The doctors still hoped that he would pull round, even at the cost of being chronically ill for the rest of his life. But he lingered a few weeks, withdrawing further and further into his illness. At last, it became necessary for him to have by-pass surgery, a long and skilful operation. He never regained consciousness. The hepatic coma lasted a fortnight, during which time he'd had a stroke, and then his body was invaded by infection – of the lungs and kidneys – and he died.

When I'd first heard he was ill, I'd offered to God that I would accept not recovering if Paul could stay alive. God wasn't interested in bargaining. Paul died and I am a great deal worse. Then again, several weeks before Paul died, my cat Polly died, apparently, of an arterial haemorrhage. She was only six and the similarity between the cause of her death and Paul's illness led me to the fanciful supposition that she had died in his place. I was wrong. I had to return to Christchurch, not only with Paul dead but also with no loving and gentle companion to help me through the desolation of my days. My grief was devastating. You might imagine that my MS would have worsened in sympathy, but it didn't. Perhaps I was buoyed up by all the support I received.

It had obviously now become impossible for me to write the whole engineering history in time for the 1987 centennial celebrations. The university's information officer was given the last third of the history and I was left with the time from the beginning in 1887 until the end of the 1950s when the school left the town site and moved out to its present position in Ilam. I was lent a computer and I worked entirely from home. My typing skills were, and are, most elementary. I used three or four fingers at most, and it was only the years of piano playing that enabled me to maintain a reasonable speed. In addition, I was computer illiterate. As I have said in a poem, 'I speak pidgin computer.'

My brief had been that the book should be not too long, detailed and readable.

A friend's father-in-law crowed, 'There'll be a little engineering, a great deal of human interest and a tiny bit of poetic licence.'

'You've rumbled me,' I admitted. 'But I'm trying to get rid of the poetic licence.'

So, in that first year after Paul's death, I had to spend most days at the computer. Maybe, if I hadn't had the intellectual challenge and company of the book during that first nightmare year, I'd have gone completely to pieces. In addition, it gave structure to my days. I had been commissioned to write a book so I felt I had no choice.

Then my landlord dropped a bombshell: he was intending to sell the flat over my head. Now, as my walk was deteriorating, it was obviously not sensible for me to live much longer in a house with stairs. Yet I was most reluctant to leave. It was not just that, in my vulnerable state, a move was too threatening. It was not just that I was under too much pressure with the engineering history to be able to spare the time to look for somewhere else. Cogent as they were, these were not the reasons why I found the idea of moving so totally unthinkable. It was because, although Paul had never visited my flat, I had spoken to him on the phone from there. However tenuous, it was still a connection between us, which I wasn't ready to sever.

In my impoverished state, it was not easy to rustle up enough money for a deposit. Fortunately, I had inherited jewellery from my godmother, some of which I never wore and therefore could sell. As well, I was eligible for a Housing Corporation loan. I must confess when I was interviewed by a corporation official, I pretended, for the first and only time in my life, that the reason for the untidy clutter in my house was that I had MS. This was arrant nonsense. I am the kind of person who would come back from a walk on hills or beach carrying dried flowers, feathers, bones, shells, stones or driftwood, all of which had to go somewhere. In addition, I was new to the computer and therefore didn't trust it. Instead of editing on the screen, I was printing off endlessly. Add piles of essays waiting to be marked to all the computer paper, and you have quite a muddle. I didn't mind. It was how I lived so I was used to it. But I mendaciously adopted a pose of helplessness so that the official wouldn't refuse me a mortgage on the grounds of all my clutter. It worked.

At this time, I was extending my walk each day until, although I wouldn't have been able to manage the walk back, I could have reached my parents' house. Then my father died suddenly in his 80th year, two days after I had heard about my loan. There was nothing malignant in his dying, but it was only seven months since Paul had died and my grief for Dad was subsumed in the greater grief for my son. It's only been in recent years that I have been able to mourn for Dad, remember him lovingly and really appreciate him. But his dying made me emotionally responsible for my mother, with whom I'd always had an uneasy relationship. And, in less than nine months, I had lost to death, my son, my father and my cat. It was no wonder I never succeeded, suppose it were possible, in getting on top of the MS. Indeed, after my father died, I never again walked as far. Thereafter, I probably managed only two-thirds of the walk, and little by little, I was managing even less. I also remember, on the day of his funeral, feeling decidedly uneasy walking across my sitting room without sticks; my balance was so shaky. Normally, I didn't need sticks in the house because the confined space gave me lots of visual cues. But that day, I lurched across the room. Even walking with my legs apart, as if I had wet my pants, didn't make me feel secure enough. I was becoming more and more disabled.

Notwithstanding, I continued writing the engineering history. The publisher's deadline was the end of October 1986. But 31 October was the first anniversary of Paul's death and there was no way I was going to meet that deadline. I needed October for thinking, feeling and remembering. I brought the deadline forward to the end of September and spent the next month in unreserved mourning.

Chapter 6

It was as we came into November that I realised the emptiness of my days. Tutoring was over for the year and wouldn't start up again until the following March. I had finished the engineering history, with all its stimulus, company and structure. My friends were mostly working, or if they weren't, had unsuitable access to their homes. What was I to do to fill my days? I was faced with all this empty time. I was familiar with Thoreau's 'as if you could kill time, without injuring eternity'. I didn't want to spend my days in banal and unconstructive activity. I was truly afraid.

Then it occurred to me that, perhaps, empty time was like a chained dog that was barking threateningly. If I took the dog off its chain, the barking would cease and it would be all over me with friendliness. Maybe, I could befriend time in the same way. I needed to transform it from something inimical and threatening into something welcoming. A real Jungian precept: if a feeling bothers you, don't push it away, don't seek out distractions; instead, you stay with it until it turns around, until you transform it. So, I set myself the following discipline: unless I gave myself special permission, as when I was reading Proust's *Remembrance of Things Past*, I allowed myself to read only at mealtimes and in the evening. Otherwise, I could play the piano or stitch at the beautiful tapestry of the lady and the unicorn that Paul had given me in Melbourne. The rest of the time I sat with a biro and clipboard and waited.

Some days, all I'd do was sit but other days an image would float up into my mind. One day, I felt as if all I was doing was putting a bucket down into an empty well and there was the first line of a poem: 'My mind's deep well is stagnant'. I could then spend the rest of the day working on that image. This was another Jungian precept: find an image for what's distressing you and work with it. I think it was mainly assumed that such an image would be visual and that working on it would be drawing or painting but, although I have a good sense of colour, I can't draw to save myself and I have found working with words also has the desired effect.

Writing poetry is a very recent outlet for me. Apart from a few, undisciplined, outpourings when Guy and I split up, I hadn't tried my hand at poetry. But, after Paul died, I found poetry worked for me. Sometimes, what I wrote was just therapy, only for myself or a few friends, but even that was enough to tip loneliness into solitude. But as I persevered, especially while I was imposing the no-reading ban on myself, I found ways of expressing myself that other people could relate to, even without knowing my circumstances. In this way, and through poetry, I did manage to befriend time.

> I measure time by raindrops
> by the restructuring of a spider's web
> by a flurry of waxeyes elegant
> in olive green and white eyeliner
> foraging for food
> around the strawberry tree
>
> light laps and ripples like polished water
> and calling blackbirds resonate
> within time's boundlessness

I am describing this change in awareness as if it were achieved easily, as if all I had to do was make a decision and thereafter everything fell into place. On the contrary, it took all my courage and discipline to stay with the emptiness and not seek distractions. Some days my efforts were laughable; after all, we're very conditioned by our busy life. Months would go past and every day was a bitter struggle. I knew what was needed but I couldn't achieve the peace of mind that comes from freeing oneself from distractions. Maybe, just before bedtime, I'd get a glimpse but it would have vanished by morning and the whole process would have to begin again. I was unbearably desolate but there was nothing anyone would have been able to suggest. Looking back, I feel as if I trudged endlessly across a desert landscape with only occasional oases. It was as if I had to renew my contract with myself each morning. I suppose I could have given up; I know friends thought I was adopting draconian measures. I could have buried myself all day and every day in a book. I could have given in and acquired a television and a video. Indeed, one of my friends suggested I get a television 'to assuage my loneliness'. But I wasn't trying to assuage my loneliness; I was trying to transform it.

So, I didn't do either of those things. One, I'm stubborn. Two, I like to be able to think, at the end of the day, that I have achieved something worthwhile, even if it is only that I have rescued two bees and a ladybird from a swimming pool. In James Hillman's telling phrase, I need to convert 'events into experiences'. I was helped in that by the sort of person I am. Wittgenstein said that there are two kinds of people: those who see the ordinary as just that, ordinary, and those who see the ordinary as extraordinary. I am very much the second kind. Three, and perhaps the most important, the experience of being there in the present moment, which followed the retreat of my unpleasant symptoms after my second MS attack, had shown me so clearly how it was supposed to be. I wasn't following some half-baked theory I had read in a book. I knew how it could be and I wanted to get back to that state.

> the approach to a gateless gate
> is fraught with danger but on the far side
> crystal hours hang motionless –
> silence like evening birds
> returning settles over the mind

Somehow, I must have known that, if I persevered, I would achieve that inner silence. Improvement was so gradual. I didn't wake one morning and realise I had won out. What happened was that the bad spells, when time was dreary and claustrophobic, became further apart. Because they were still so frequent, I didn't realise that the gaps between them were getting greater. I still seemed to spend endless time fretting, full of resentment and unvoiced accusations at my friends, who didn't seem to understand, although how they could I don't know, when I neither understood myself nor shared my feelings.

I think perhaps I was ultimately helped to come to terms with all the empty time by a perception I'd had soon after learning I had multiple sclerosis. I remember thinking: I don't like this, I don't want it but now I have it, I'll have to learn to live inside it with, in my friend's phrase, dignity and grace. And I asked myself what the illness had given me. And the answer was time, time to be contemplative. I thought of the stories about men in India who, having been householders for many years, in mid-life abandoned all their material comforts and went out on the road as pilgrims. In a sense, that was what had happened to me. Sure, I couldn't be a travelling pilgrim, but, for all that, I had to live my life as a traveller. I was definitely journeying into uncharted territory. I liked the fact that, undertaking my own Pilgrim's Progress, I lived in Bunyan Street. I don't believe God has given me this condition, but, in some obscure way, I feel it has been asked of me to deal with it honourably.

A friend once asked me an unexpected question: 'Are you committed to the illness?' Later, when I asked him what had prompted the enquiry, he couldn't for the life of him remember ever having asked it, or even wanting to ask it. But I remember very clearly the answer I gave him, an answer that would fit no other question: 'I am not committed to the illness, but to the way of life that goes with it'.

Chapter 7

So, I had, more or less, dealt with my changed life in psychological/spiritual terms. But, all that time, the physical deterioration had not ceased. I was out of remission; the MS was rampaging, it was seeping and creeping. I kept having to come up with new strategies. Has it ever occurred to you to wonder how a person walking with two sticks copes with carrying anything, especially anything as potentially dangerous as a hot cup of tea? I lived, at that time, in an ownership flat with a hatch between the small kitchen and the sitting room. The only problem was that I wanted to drink my cup of tea on the far side of the room, by the windows, where I had a good view of the neighbour's sycamore trees. Also, the bird feeder was in the courtyard. The trouble was I had the whole stretch of room to cross. I took to putting the cup of tea on the hatch on a tray, coming round to sit on a chair by the hatch, putting the tray and myself on floor and shuffling us both over to the window, putting the tray on my stool, then standing up so that I could sit in my armchair, pick up the tray and drink my cuppa. It was a time-consuming, not entirely agreeable activity that I had to repeat several times a day. Thoroughly fed up with the whole rigmarole, I asked my occupational therapist for advice. 'You need a wheelchair,' she maintained.

Now, I was living in a house with stairs. The bedroom, study, bathroom and lavatory were all upstairs. This was before the days when I had a commode downstairs, so I was struggling up the stairs half a dozen times a day. The woman was out of her mind, or rather she was manifesting a trait I often came up against, of going right to the final solution without checking out any intermediary solutions. Needless to say, I rejected her suggestion. Before I solved it in my own way, I asked around. Sons of a friend suggested I needed either a long straw or a skateboard. I could always have put the drink in a thermos and then in a bag round my neck but I opted in the end for an attractive cane trolley with heavy glass shelves. That meant it was quite stable, unlike the ones that ran at the lightest push, no use at all to someone off balance. I could walk quite confidently with it. And it wasn't an eyesore. I put lots of pretty things on it and sometimes, Fox, the new cat I had acquired six months after Polly died, would sit on it.

That was one problem dealt with. Another, of course, was the stairs, a lethal trap. And, to make matters worse, the piano was right next to the foot of the stairs so that I risked cracking my head open on it if I fell. So I took to sitting down at the top and coming down on my bottom, like a toddler. I found if I stopped two steps from the foot of the stairs with my feet on the carpet, I could pull myself to an upright position; the cane trolley was always parked at the bottom of the stairs for me to grab as soon as I was standing. Increasingly, I was using the trolley for support instead of using sticks, or later, elbow crutches in the house. My method of coming down the stairs attracted a good deal of amusement. Occasionally, a friend from the choir I had joined came visiting with his two pre-school age children. They'd show me that they could come downstairs on their tummies. I'd point out that I was longer than they were. Their father told me they'd say to him, 'Let's go and see the lady who comes down the stairs on her bottom.' So, in my small way, I had become famous.

Another difficulty I encountered was cutting things, onions or Fox's ox heart, for example. I held onto the bench with one hand and grasped the onion with the other, but then there was the knife as well. I needed at least three hands. Eventually, I acquired a padded kitchen chair and a large piece of wood that fitted across one of the drawers. That way, I could sit sideways on and fit my knees under the drawer. But before I organised this set-up, I used to cut up food sitting on the floor. If it was ox heart Fox would sit beside me and receive each chunk as I cut it. He certainly approved of the technique.

But the occupational therapist disapproved completely. Apparently, it was not in her books that a middle-aged woman could sit on the floor to perform such a task. I found her reaction ridiculously conventional. When you're disabled, one of the things you need to dispense with straight away, is convention. You're not going to be able to do things the way you used to or the way everyone else does them. You're going to need to cultivate lateral thinking. Do I need to do this at all? Is there any other way I can do it? Are there any aids I can get that will help me to do it? If you're going to bother about convention or the right way to do something, you may end up handicapping yourself far more than is necessary.

In the year after Paul's death, I started going to an indoor swimming pool once a week at a time when they offered a session for the disabled. At first, I could still manage breaststroke but, after a while, I could do only dog paddle. I found the swim gave me valuable exercise, so I looked around for other pools. I much prefer to swim outdoors under the sky; the chlorine dissipates and the temperature of the water is usually lower, which I prefer. It's more invigorating and, anyway, MS doesn't like warmth. I was especially lucky in living very close to two outdoor pools: a public pool, the Waltham Lido, which is slightly heated, and the small pool of the Waltham primary school, totally unheated. I rented a key to the school pool and over two summers I'd swim most days. Sometimes, the water was so cold that my forehead would go numb, despite my not putting my head under. I suppose I was taking a risk swimming in such cold water on my own, but I found it refreshing. The worst of it was that I couldn't get in quickly; I had to sit on the top of the stone steps and lower myself down on my bottom: talk about pulling the sticking plaster off slowly. I had never been a fast or showy swimmer, but I was a very confident one. I had been well taught after I had jumped, before I could swim, into deep water after my five years older brother. He was doing it, so I could see no reason why I shouldn't be able to as well. They fished me out and my mother made immediate arrangements for me to take swimming lessons; obviously I wasn't traumatised, as I have no fear of the water.

After a couple of years, though, I found the walk from the gate of the school pool to the steps just too much – walking back presented no difficulty, as my body functioned better for an hour or so after the swim. I then transferred my summer swims to the Lido. I have been very fortunate in the pool attendants who, for many years, let me swim on weekdays before the pool opened to the public, while they were cleaning it. At one stage also, at weekends, several people used to swim earlier than the public hours and I was able to join this select côterie.

As well, over the winter, two or three times a week, I went to an inside pool. It was mainly for serious swimmers doing their training, but there was a slow lane for people like me. I gave myself, and the attendants of that pool, a great fright one day. I used to park close to the glass doors at the entrance, so that I didn't have as far to walk to reach the changing room for the disabled. On this day, as I was entering the car park, some little thing about how I negotiated myself into position was different and I had to make an unexpected movement of my foot from brake to accelerator and back to brake. My foot wouldn't lift and I drove slowly, but inexorably, into the glass doors. All that was in my mind was an immense panic that, if the doors didn't stop me, I'd drive into the pool. I did stop in time, however, embarrassed and distressed. The pool officials were very kind and gentle with me, glad, as the receptionist said, that it was only doors I'd damaged and not me or anyone else. As there were often toddlers at the pool for water safety classes, she had a very good point.

Utterly shaken by the event, I rehearsed it over and over in my mind. At first, I thought to myself, well, I know how it happened and I can make sure it doesn't happen again. That is what I do in other circumstances. If I fall because I have placed my walking stick or elbow crutch on a piece of paper that slips away from me, taking the stick and me with it, I can learn from what I have done so that I don't do again. But then it occurred to me that, when it was a driving accident, there was more at stake than whether I managed not to fall. I was putting my own, and others', lives at risk. When I had bought the car, hand controls, unattached, had been included. I arranged for my local garage to install them. But they were unworkable. The brake was either full on or full off; there was no slowing down capacity. I complained to the garage, but the man who'd installed them claimed he had found no problem. After all, I was a woman *and* disabled. Of course, I must be wrong.

Feeling rather desperate, I found a firm that specialised in car modifications. One of their mechanics came and fetched my car and drove it to the workshop. After he tried the hand controls, he agreed with me: I had no slowing capacity. The new ones he installed were much more satisfactory. For a few years, I drove using the foot accelerator and the hand control brake. When my hand automatically sought the hand control brake if I drove past a dog or a young child on a bicycle, I knew I'd adapted totally to hand controls.

Eventually, though, I could no longer manage the foot accelerator. I could depress it, but I couldn't ease off or remove my foot entirely when I was braking. That meant I was accelerating and braking simultaneously. I doubted whether it was safe and, anyway, I didn't think it would be doing my engine much good. So, I learnt to use the hand accelerator. I can't say I enjoyed driving as much as I had, but at least I was still moderately independent.

The indoor swimming pool staff were greatly relieved when I turned up for my next swim and assured them that now I had hand controls and their glass doors were safe from me in the future. For a while, I was able to keep up winter swims, but, eventually the walk in from the car became too much and I would have needed too much help getting dressed and undressed, so I had to give them up.

I had acquired a motorised scooter and that meant I could, at least, still manage to get to the Lido in the summer, although, increasingly, I needed two people to lift me in and out: a pool attendant and a friend, helper or attendant carer. I found, as well, after a few years that, when I was dog paddling, I could no longer hold my head up high enough to avoid breathing in copious amounts of water. The problem was that I couldn't stay all the time on my back; I needed to be on my front to turn at the end of my width. I preferred widths to lengths because I had great trouble swimming straight; with widths, I was right next to the side, could see it and that kept me straighter. Eventually, I solved the problem of the turn by swimming, as I reached the edge, on my front with my head under and my eyes open so I could gauge where I was. This, however, did mean my eyes became very itchy from the chlorine.

I'm describing all this in the past tense because, last summer, I managed a mere half dozen swims; I have deteriorated to the point where I can manage only with an attendant carer. I need someone to be in the water with me at the beginning; until I've been in the pool a while, I swim very tentatively. In fact, it would be truer to say that I don't really swim at all; my carer walks beside me, towing me on my back for the first width. I also need her to check out that I can manage the turns, both at the side of the pool and, in the middle, from my front to my back. Once I am confident that, for this swim at least, the turns are all right, my companion can swim without worrying about me. Considering I used to swim most days even in dubious weather – I can remember one attendant calling out to me as I swam up and down in the rain, 'Don't get wet!' – I miss the swims sorely. I wasn't comfortable in the water – my sensory nerves are too damaged – but I enjoyed the exercise, I benefited from the increased oxygen and I'd gain a great sense of achievement. Despite the fact that all the odds were stacked against me, I was still managing.

About two years into the MS rampage, my kind brother-in-law and his wife paid for me to go privately to a neurologist. I don't know what they hoped this would achieve, but, in the event, he told me my walk was affected and my hands were starting to deteriorate also. That cost $180. I could have told him that. If I had, would he have given me $180?

The only thing I gained was the suggestion that I might find an exercycle useful. I duly acquired one and added two brief sessions of exercycling to my daily yoga, meditation and yoga breathing routine. When it became too difficult to climb on and off, I acquired an arrangement that I could use while I was still sitting in my comfortable chair. But even that got beyond me, when I gave myself third-degree burns in 1996 and had such thick bandages that I couldn't fit my feet into stirrups. Once the bandages were off, I tried again but my calf muscles had diminished too much. MS is a memory fault. I have found over and over that if, for some reason, I can no longer do a movement, unless I pick it up again really quickly, it has gone for ever.

I can offer several examples. During the burnt feet episode, I lost a yoga pose, *Supta Virasana*, where I first sat with my knees bent back so that my feet were right next to my body, then I lay back in the same position with my arms stretched over my head. This was a wonderful stretch for the thighs and trunk. When the feet healed a little, I tried it again but my thigh muscles protested vigorously. I thought at first that this was just a temporary problem so I persevered but the pain in my thighs has persisted. I soon realised I couldn't attempt the pose on my own as the pain would shoot my legs out of the position in a vicious spasm. After 27 years of doing the pose daily, my body has forgotten what to do.

Again, it had got to the stage where the only time I walked with elbow crutches was in the nearby park. At home, I had the trolley or the walls and I tended to use my shower stool as a walking frame; the legs splayed out and made it very stable.

Most days I walked a short distance in the park between a double row of sycamores. The trees gave me visual cues telling me where I was in space and, from time to time, I stopped and tightened my knees until I could feel the skin stretch, another cue to position me in space so that I wouldn't fall over. It was a very short walk, no more than a cricket pitch distance from the scooter and back. On two separate occasions, total strangers driving past the park, stopped to ask me whether I needed help. Seeing me walking away from the scooter made them assume it had broken down and my precarious progress made them anxious for me. This is just one of many instances of the kindness I have received in these years since I have been visibly disabled.

This particular year, 1992, we had a very, and continuously, wet winter. I found walking in the park too difficult because of all the mud that would cling to my shoes and the tips of my elbow crutches. I kept up my limited walk by thumping my way around on concrete near the garage with a shower stool. When the weather brightened and the ground became less muddy, I found I could no longer walk with elbow crutches. My balance just wasn't good enough. A few weeks before the rainy time had started, my physio had come to watch me walk in the park. She was most impressed, as she didn't think I could possibly manage to walk without more support. Sadly, a few months later, she was right.

The same problem of losing a skill, because I haven't been able to practise it, has happened with my driving. An auto-electrician kept my car for several months and when, at last, I got it back, I found I had lost the necessary, unthinking habits associated with driving. It has been said that I have lost my nerve but it is a physical not a psychological problem. I have also lost a great deal of function in my left hand and arm. With hand controls, the onus of steering the car rests almost entirely on the left arm. I can hook my right thumb over the steering wheel when accelerating, but if I am braking I have to push the control away from me and, therefore, steer entirely with my left arm. If you consider that I'm off balance anyway so that cornering is, in itself, difficult, you will understand that I don't feel safe driving. Any time I need to brake, which includes going round corners, I have to rely on an unsafe left arm. If I've lost my nerve, there may well be other drivers who are glad to hear it.

Chapter 8

It was not long after I came out of remission at the beginning of 1985 that I had to face up to the problem of how I was to present myself to strangers now that I was visibly disabled. When I first started walking round the university on sticks, it was the skiing season. People just assumed I had had a skiing accident, so I was only occasionally asked about my disability. The question would be 'What have you done?' not 'What is the matter?' Adults, anyway, are usually reticent about asking; the children I encountered in the park when I was walking with my clumsy gait were more forthcoming. Even so, their parents would shush them as if they had been rude. I much prefer a child's directness, which acknowledges the reality of my situation. When an adult supposedly protects me by maintaining a studied silence, it feels as if they're protecting themselves, which only confirms me in my isolation. Yet it's a fine line. People say, 'But I don't think of you as disabled.' That is partly saying that I am far more than my damaged body; I have a heart and soul and mind. But it is also saying, 'I don't want to have to admit you're as bad as you are. I find it threatening, although I'd never own up to that.' The truth is that, no matter how people choose to overlook it, I am disabled. It's like living with an elderly great-aunt who has constantly to be taken into account. It is she who is fidgety and restless, constantly changing position. If it were not for her, I would have lived a very different life.

At the time of my coming out of remission, I was still tutoring at the University of Canterbury. Each year, in March, I would have to introduce myself to some 50 new students. Tutorials always started about the time of the equinox, when Canterbury is particularly prone to nor'west winds. MS is notoriously uncomfortable with nor'westers: they create more positive ions, which have a dire effect on the nervous system. They make the signals take longer to get through. I am always painfully aware, in a nor'wester, that this is how bad I really am. Anyway, come the first tutorials, I'd lurch in on my elbow crutches to be greeted by the shocked faces of my first-year students. 'What on earth have we got here?' It was as if an enormous chasm had opened up between us. I was their teacher, responsible for them; it was, therefore, up to me to provide a bridge over the chasm. I needed to persuade them to laugh with me, not at me. I came up with various throwaway lines.

'I've got multiple sclerosis but it's got my legs, not my tongue.' I meant that I didn't have slurred speech, not that I was acerbic.

'I've got multiple sclerosis but I've got naturally curly hair and it's a great responsibility.'

And they'd laugh.

Later, when I had progressed from a motorised scooter to a wheel-chair, my first tutorials fell two weeks after I'd got the wheelchair. Electric wheelchairs are very hard to drive until you've got used to them, and mine, an unusual model, has only three wheels, which makes it even harder. I wibble-wobbled into my first class while the students looked on in horror.

'I can assure you,' I said with dignity, 'that I know more about teaching than I do about driving an electric wheelchair.'

Again, they laughed. Some weeks later, I pointed out that I was managing much better and they applauded.

Back then, also, I used to have to stand and stretch regularly to ease the spastic tightness of my leg muscles – I won't take anti-spasm medi-cation – so I'd tell them it would be worse if I said 'Um' at the end of every sentence. After all, I could talk or listen just as well when I was standing. It was only reading out loud that was impossible. One year, students told me at the end of the course that they no longer noticed my doing it, although I was stretching every few minutes.

I think they found a tutor on elbow crutches more alarming than a tutor on a motorised scooter. Although, actually it meant that I was worse, it looked as if I were more in control, much less as if I were going to have to be picked up from the floor any minute.

By and large, I have found students, and indeed people in general, enormously kind and helpful. I have particularly noticed men of all ages going out of their way to be caring. I have come to wonder whether this is a disregarded aspect of men's nature. Before I became disabled, I was probably too high-powered to encounter, or indeed, invite such kindness. But now I greatly appreciate it. Even small boys have evinced concern and generosity for my situation. In the days when I was still walking, I would often have a conversation with a four-year-old who played in the park with his German shepherd. He was always troubled at my slow and awkward progress. Then there came the day when he said that he'd like to lend me his legs for five minutes so that I could run. I found this the most delightful offer, an example of the splendid unself-consciousness of children.

Presenting myself in a jokey way has paid off in other ways. I remember struggling down a plane gangway with several airport staff watching. Because the steps were metal, I didn't fancy coming down them on my bottom as I did at home and as I had done at our small local theatre. Falling onto the tarmac did not appeal to me so I was coming down very gingerly.

'I wish to make it known publicly,' I declared vehemently, 'I am not drunk.'

All the attendants laughed. I surprised myself as much as the staff. I had not planned to say this; it just came out. The clown stance I had adopted had become second nature.

On occasions, moving me is unusually difficult. When I am lifted into the swimming pool the sudden shock of the cool water on my sensory nerves, especially if it's a hot day, can induce a corpse spasm, where my whole body goes rigid as if it is suffering from *rigor mortis*. I have found myself saying, 'I do this on purpose to draw attention to myself.' This is usually greeted with laughter.

Another throwaway line came as a result of what one of the young women in my choir once said. 'Diana,' she admonished me, 'stop saying you're sorry you're a nuisance.'

How right she was! And here was me, the bossy one, the one a friend pleaded with once not to go to an assertiveness training course, the one who advised the Multiple Sclerosis Society that any woman diagnosed with MS should forthwith enrol at such a course, here I was falling into the victim trap. I acknowledged the pertinence of her rebuke. Now I say, 'I've been told I'm not to keep on saying I'm sorry I'm a nuisance, so I'll say I'm glad I'm a nuisance.'

The only drawback of putting on a clown mask to facilitate my dealings with others is that it has now become so much a part of me that I never take it off. There was one afternoon, a year or so ago, when I'd had such difficulty placing my legs in an appropriate yoga pose that I cried aloud in misery, 'I can't bear it.' At that moment, the phone rang. It was a friend with a grumble about incipient flu. Did I tell her how I was feeling? No! I commiserated and then returned to my interrupted yoga practice.

Other ways of responding to my condition also became second nature, so much so that I would even hear a voice in my head making comments to me. This is how it came about. In one of our London yoga classes, Silva, Iyengar's second in command, instructed us that, though we might not always be able to change our circumstances, we could always change our attitude to them. She was directing this towards a woman in the class whose husband had just started dallying with a much younger woman. I was very much struck with the cogency of this remark and took it on board.

When I have a fall, because of my not knowing where I am in space, together with damaged sensory nerves which tend to exaggerate what I am feeling, I have no way of knowing how much I am hurt. Initially, my mind is full of panic. On one occasion the voice in my head admonished me severely: 'That's enough of that! Now see what you've done to yourself.' As it turned out, I hadn't done myself any harm; it was the strangeness and unfamiliarity of the position that had unsettled me.

Another time, the voice in my head was even more adamant. It was a hot nor'west day and I'd driven to the park for my short daily walk under the trees. When I returned, I knew I couldn't risk putting the car back in the garage. My balance, or rather, lack of it, just wouldn't cope with the open space I'd have to negotiate before I could reach the fence and hang on. So, I parked outside my gate. Unfortunately, there was not only no culvert but also a very deep gutter. I tried unsuccessfully to get across it but, after several attempts, I gave up. I had no choice but to sit on the pavement, swing my legs over the gutter, stand up and totter inside. At first, I collapsed into a chair, quite overcome with distress, then the voice in my head said quite clearly, 'What's all the fuss about? You wanted to get into the house and you did, even if by a rather unorthodox method. At least, it wasn't pouring with rain, when the gutter would have been desperately flooded. Now, ring the city council and arrange for a culvert.'

I meekly did as I was told. I had indoctrinated myself into changing my attitude.

One of the very real difficulties of a neurological illness, or condition, as I prefer to call it, is explaining it to people. If you say you have flu, a sore back or a headache, everyone understands what you mean. But if you say you send a signal to your foot to lift off the floor and the foot ignores it, it is harder to comprehend. Walking is automatic once you're out of your toddler days. So, I've had to come up with metaphors – a puppet, a disagreeable husband – although finding suitable metaphors doesn't always work. I told a friend once that it was as if I had prickly heat. Ignoring the 'as if', she recommended putting baking soda in my bath water!

I once asked my physio whether I could have a fall and end up in a bizarre position that I couldn't get out of, so that I'd be there till someone came. She said, 'Yes!' I knew I was living with a great deal of risk, but, for a while, I chose not to get an alarm. I decided I'd wait until the disaster had struck.

There were, however, various near misses. One morning I was getting out of bed when something made me tip backwards. I was now lying back with my feet on the floor. In such a position, I need to be able to haul myself upright by pulling on something. The only available lever, the edge of my bedside table, was out of reach. So, too, therefore, was the phone. I was well and truly stuck. It was a Sunday and I had no certainty of any visitor until the following evening. Unless I came up with a solution, I would be there for around 36 hours. I didn't fancy it. So, I squirmed and wriggled for about 10 minutes, until, at last, I managed to tip myself on to the floor. Then I had to slide myself along on my bottom, pulling the shower stool to the top of the stairs where, with difficulty I could stand up, turn around and thump my way back to the bedroom. The whole exercise had taken 20 minutes.

After that fright, I had an arrangement with a neighbour that I would ring her at the same time every day. If I didn't, she would ring me. If there was no answer, she was to come and check me out – she knew where the key was hidden. This meant that the longest I could be undiscovered was 24 hours and, as I used to ring her at 4.30 p.m., just before I started my daily yoga practice, and I was always better from then till bedtime, I was really only at risk for eight hours or so.

My next disaster had me ringing a friend at 8 o'clock each morning. By then, I had a cordless phone that went everywhere with me. One evening I slipped getting off the exercycle and ended up with one foot jammed so that I couldn't wriggle free. But I could reach the phone to summon help, so I wasn't there very long. The friend who arranged my morning call seemed most anxious that I wouldn't make it down the stairs. But, actually, first thing was not when I was most at risk. My most precarious time has always been after lunch. My temperature rises each day about 2 p.m. and as MS does not like heat, my symptoms are noticeably worse mid-afternoon.

When I moved to my present house in 1993, these arrangements were, somehow, discontinued. It must have seemed as if I were less at risk because the house lacked stairs. This wasn't so, however.

The next disaster occurred some years after I had shifted to my present house. I had had my mattress turned; it is an inner-spring mattress and the new side, previously unused, behaved just like a trampoline. Around 5 a.m. one morning, my feet had wriggled their way out of the bed. I woke, as often happened, to find them cold and purple, hanging down off the bed. I had to sit up before I could hoist them, with difficulty because they had become heavy with spasticity, back into bed. As I sat up, the mattress trampolined me onto the floor. I fell so that I was leaning back against the wheelchair with my head on the seat. I was not madly uncomfortable and, as it was early April, it was not particularly cold. The trouble was that, in that position, I needed to have something to pull on to bring me upright. The bedside table where the cordless phone was charging was out of reach. It was a Sunday and I knew a friend was dropping in at some time during the day but I didn't know when. It might not be until mid-afternoon. There was no way I wanted to stay where I was for 10 hours or so. Apart from anything else, I need to change my position every 5 to 10 minutes to ease the spasticity. Maybe this was the situation the physio had warned me of. I said out loud to my body, 'If you don't show me what to do, we'll be here for too long.'

Then it came to me to wriggle myself sideways until I was lying on the floor. I expected to end up lying parallel to the wheelchair and would then have had to work myself, little by little, around until I could reach the table and the phone. To my great surprise I found myself lying at right angles to the wheelchair. It was a matter of seconds to pull the table leg towards me, reach the phone and dial for help. While I waited for the help to arrive, I was able to do my yoga breathing. Another near disaster had been averted. The friend came at 2.30, so I could have been there for nine and a half hours.

I had been living with a great deal of risk. In the end, about two years ago, for all that I am, as my doctor has said, 'fiercely independent',

I realised the risk factor had become unacceptably high and I gave in and got myself connected to one of those security alarm systems. I have a chain round my neck and I have to press a medallion. A message goes through to a computer; I am rung to check that my call for help is genuine. If it is, someone comes to see what's wrong. I may have to wait up to 20 or 30 minutes, but someone does come in the end.

Last year, however, I fell in the bathroom when my phone was off the hook. The security people kept getting the engaged signal when they rang and assumed I was talking to a friend and, therefore, all right, even though I kept pressing my alarm gadget. I knew they were ringing me, because I was lying there, all scrumpled, listening to the engaged beeps. Luckily, someone was due in half an hour. She put the phone back on the hook and a security man was round in five minutes to help her lift me off the floor. He promptly changed my access so that, in future, it can be ascertained whether I'm talking or the phone is off the hook. If the problem was going to happen, it was well that it did so on a day when I was expecting a visitor. That meant I was only on the floor for 35 minutes, which was a great help, especially as there really wasn't room for me to fall and I was in a rather uncomfortable reef knot.

Chapter 9

After 1985 my condition slowly, but inexorably, deteriorated. I had reached the point where I did very little walking in the house, except when I was upstairs. And the stairs themselves had become a major problem. It was a pity I couldn't go up them on my bottom the way I came down. I had tried and, although I could manage one step, a whole flight was beyond me. To walk upstairs, I had to lift a foot up and then bring it forward, in two separate movements. Increasingly, gravity was getting me, so that I couldn't lift the foot high enough, or even at all, and if I could, then I couldn't also lift it forward. I found it more difficult in the afternoon, when, because of my circadian temperature changes, all the MS symptoms were worse. It was also harder on hot nor'west days. At first, I was still determined to stay in the flat, and, to that end, I borrowed a commode with a view to having a second lavatory installed downstairs. The commode meant I had to go upstairs only twice a day: once in the morning, after I had meditated, to have a shower, and again at bedtime.

But, in the end, it became obvious that I was living in cloud-cuckoo-land. The changes that would be necessary to make the flat wheelchair friendly were just too extreme. So, reluctantly, I decided to look for somewhere else to live. I wanted to stay in the same district for a variety of reasons: I liked being near the river and the hills; I liked being near a little park and swimming pool; I had several neighbours I could call on for help, which, at this stage, was nothing more serious than Fox bringing in a live sparrow.

At first, the chances of my finding something close by seemed rather remote. However, there was a little old lady in a house opposite the park, who told me she'd hurt her foot falling off her bike. For a few weeks I sat like a turkey vulture on her fence, willing her to decide she'd have to go into care. But before that happened I registered that a large house in a large garden diagonally opposite me on one corner of the park was up for sale, and that I actually knew the place. In fact, its occupants had been very helpful in the matter of Fox and the sparrows.

But for some reason, perhaps because it was so big, I hadn't given it a thought. Then one day, I was sitting doing yoga when I thought, 'Why not?' I rang the estate agent, went through the house with friends the next day and the following day made an offer which was accepted. I had just become the owner of a large house – three or four bedrooms, two living rooms, one small and one very big, and a sunroom – set in a very well-established quarter-acre section. The garden is a lovely mix of natives – kowhai, five finger, pittosporum, ake-ake, flax, rimu and native beech – and flowering deciduous trees: azalea, japonica, lilac, rhododendron, floribunda crab-apple, ornamental cherry and double cherry. As well, there are lots of fruit trees, a walnut and a massive grapevine. Because of all the trees, it is very enclosed and private; indeed, it has the feeling of a sanctuary. After having had only a very small courtyard shaded by a neighbour's sycamore trees, I could hardly believe my luck. I hadn't realised how starved I was for such natural beauty. In the first week after I moved in, I sat outside more than I had in the previous four years. In the past, when I was still well, I had gained much strength by sitting looking at sea and sky or hills and sky. Now once more, I can nourish my roots by spending long hours looking at trees and sky.

> showered by autumn gold
> I stand alone at leaf fall –
> it feels like a bridal –
> here in the presence of witnesses
> red and white roses standing sentinel
> a smoke bush burning against the sky
> a little cat dappled with light
> I take this garden
> in sunlight and in shadow
> for better for worse

A man I knew slightly, who used to write tree and garden articles for the *Press*, told a friend, 'Diana has bought a garden.' The house, it appears, was of no account.

In the last month in the old place, I had a fortnight's visit from my four-year-old godson, his mother and elder sister. Now, a pocket handkerchief-sized courtyard does not provide much playing space.

Fortunately, my sparrow-rescuing friends had already shifted to their new house, leaving their university student son in possession of my new house. He was hardly ever home and didn't mind at all if my friend and I brought the children over to play in the garden. That was a specially good idea, as it turned out, since Fox always followed us over and, in that way, became used to the garden before the actual move.

The house is a 1920s bungalow with some of the original features such as rimu wood panelling in hall and sitting room. Any modifications, for example enlarged windows, have been done very tastefully. The kitchen and bathroom have been brought up to date and sport modern rimu panelling. The only room with carpet is the small sitting room; all the remaining rooms have polished rimu floors. When the occupational therapist came to see what modifications were needed, she looked in delight at both house and garden.

'Don't you let anyone tell you it's too big,' she admonished. 'It's almost your entire world.'

I am very aware of this now that I am house- and garden-bound. I may be in a prison, but it is a very beautiful prison, with lots of variety.

It didn't need too many modifications. The ramp is wooden and I paid the extra amount to have the wooden porch onto which it abutted painted the same olive green, so that the ramp is less intrusive. In fact, it looked so much as if it belonged that I was congratulated on being so sensible as to buy a house with a ramp. Other modifications were to the bathroom. A wet floor area was installed, the lavatory was eventually raised and rails were put in beside it. The house has two lavatories, one in a little room off the wash-house. I was lucky in that this was an old house with the main lavatory in the bathroom. This has made it much more accessible, although it could be better situated. And, it being an old house, the floor slopes, which means there is often a flood after a shower, especially if I have brought in a leaf on my wheelchair tyres.

Moving was easy. There was no need to get a removal van. Friends rallied round and trudged backwards and forwards across the road with wheelbarrow loads of plants and books. The previous owner produced a trolley for the piano. I rang out for pizzas and we all had lunch on the lawn. By evening, everything was in place, if not in its final position. My desktop computer and stereo had been set up, books, even if half of them were upside down, were on the shelves, and the kitchen things were away, although many in high cupboards I couldn't reach. In the next few days, apart from sitting in the garden, there was a lot of rationalisation to be got through. I had really loved the flat and was sad to be leaving it. After all, it had supported me through great distress; it had been the companion of my grieving. But, in the end, I came over here without a backward glance. My new house fitted me like a glove. From the very first day, I felt I completely belonged. It is a house that has been much loved and its atmosphere is healing. I would like to live here till I die.

In practical terms, what I missed most when I shifted, strangely, was the stairs. It had got to the stage where I couldn't stand up if I was sitting on the floor. Originally, to get up from the floor, I used to kneel, then curl my toes round so I could balance myself on my hands and feet, then I'd need to hang onto something to haul myself upright. But I often couldn't manage that. Instead, I had to bump myself across the room on my bottom and heave myself into a sitting position on the bottom step. Then, at last, and it used to take ages, I could stand up.

But now that I had shifted, I had to devise another way of standing up after yoga or if I fell. I gave it some thought and, at last, hit upon an idea. First I had to place the stool strategically beside my comfy chair. If I knelt beside the stool, I could then sit on it. After an astute wriggle, I could transfer myself to the chair. The whole exercise took 5 to 10 minutes. It was also dependent on the height of the chair remaining the same. Yet, as I deteriorated further, it was getting harder and harder to stand up from my chair. It wouldn't be long before I needed the chair put up on blocks; this would alter the relative proportion of stool to chair. Such a method of getting up from the floor, therefore, was only a temporary expedient.

For all that, I managed in this way for a year or so; once I even had to bump myself on my bottom all the way from the bathroom to the sitting room after I'd had a fall. But then, it just became too difficult. When I'd had to ring for help in getting up off the floor after yoga three times in one week, I realised it was time to come up with another strategy. After all, it was all very well bothering neighbours and friends if I'd had a fall. It was altogether different when I'd put myself down on the floor deliberately, and seven times a week at that. To give up yoga was quite unthinkable. I had to find some solution.

In the end, I had the mattress removed from the spare bed and a piece of hardboard nailed across it somewhat wider than the, admittedly very narrow, bed. I had first tried doing yoga on the mattress itself but I rapidly discovered I needed a harder surface. While I could still stand, provided I had something to hold onto, getting on and off the bed posed no problem. When such standing transfers became impossible, I had to resort to sliding transfers. By then, I had been allocated, as I mentioned earlier, a rather nippy wheelchair. Because it has only three wheels, it is a great deal more manoeuvrable than the four-wheeled variety. The other important aspect of this wheelchair is that it has a hydraulic device, which means it can be raised and lowered. In this way, now that I have to resort to sliding transfers, I can raise the wheelchair to accommodate what ever I am sliding onto – bed, chair, shower stool, lavatory – instead of having to get all these items raised. So I found I could slide on and off the bed on which I did yoga without having to bother neighbours. For now, my yoga was safe.

I practise each day for approximately one hour, even if I now manage only three or four poses. Twice a week, I have special help from a young friend who comes in to assist me with two more difficult poses – the one I mentioned earlier when I lie back with my knees bent and my feet by my side, and a version of a shoulder stand where I have my thighs on a chair that is placed over my head. In the first minutes of my practice, I can feel a change in my energy levels; it's like a flat battery being charged or a slow puncture mended. Tiredness is a major MS symptom that I have never suffered from. Oh yes, I can get tired if I overdo it, but I don't start off the day tired. Rather, I can feel as if my overload has gone. My parents lived in an old house, where the electricity would cut off if too many power outlets were used. This meant that their overload had gone. All that was needed, however, was to unplug something and turn a special switch and power was restored. I lack that special switch although, over the years, yoga has come very close to providing it.

My life in the new house changed only a little. On fine days, I spend several hours in my garden, growing into the lawn like the trees. An existing structure outside was converted into an aviary in which I have canaries. About a year ago, a second cat, called Orlando because, at first, I didn't know what sex she was, adopted us, much to Fox's chagrin. I regard the aviary as their television set and, since there are field mice in there too, as one of my friends has said, 'They've got two channels.'

Then, six months ago at my gardener's suggestion, I acquired a half wine barrel with water plants, initially four, but now only three, fish and an undisclosed number of water snails. I have a bird feeder and my garden is excellent for blackbirds and waxeyes, so there's always a great deal going on. Sometimes, I write a poem in my head about some aspect of my garden, which I then write down when I come inside. My verbal memory means that if I just keep repeating the words over and over, they become transfixed in my memory.

Now that I have befriended time, I no longer need to adopt the draconian no-reading-until-the-evening measures. I feel free to read whenever I want to. But the habit of just sitting, doing nothing and waiting, has become so entrenched that I can feel sideways with myself if I have too much company or too many distractions. I may have given in and acquired a television, but all I watch are videos, at the moment *Brideshead Revisited.* As well, writing poetry is a contemplative exercise. I may sit a whole day and not write anything at all, but the only reason I do write something the following day is because of the long previous silence.

Chapter 10

It is really the keenness of my response to the world about me that has kept me, so far, off anti-spasm medication. At one stage, early on, the doctor, who wanted to feel he was helping, offered me some.

'What are the side effects?' I asked.

'Sleepiness,' he replied.

'You can keep it,' I assured him.

It seemed to me then, as it still does, that all I have left is the quality of my mind. I have no intention of muddying that, if I can possibly help it. And, after all, at that time I was only extremely uncomfortable, not in absolute pain. And, despite that discomfort, I was still able to get to sleep. Not brilliantly, and I did, and still do, snooze a little during the day if I'm especially warm because of the sun or heater, but when you need to change position every few minutes, that's not really a good idea. So, I continued to resist taking anti-spasm.

There came another time when I must have complained to the doctor rather more than usual, and, in a fit of weakness – perhaps I felt sorry for his helplessness in the face of my usual intransigence – I allowed him to prescribe valium, which is also used as an anti-spasm. The chemist's boy delivered it and I put it in the kitchen cupboard while I considered what to do. The next day I still hadn't made up my mind whether to take it or not. I sat that afternoon looking out at the sunshine on the sycamore trees – I was still living in the ownership flat – when I became aware of a magical quality of light. Now, this is not unknown in Canterbury on a cloudy nor'west day. Then, there is always an arch over the mountains to the west and in late afternoon, when the setting sun drops below the arch, the light is always incredible. But this was mid-afternoon on a clear day with an easterly blowing. I have also usually found it to be the case that when I experience something unusual, like this luminous light, it disappears as soon as I describe it to myself in words. But this light didn't disappear. On the contrary, it lasted long enough for me to write a poem in my head.

Needless to say, the pills stayed in the cupboard and were ultimately flushed down the lavatory. I felt as if I had had a clear directive. After all, I have all these years of yoga and meditation behind me. The Buddhists describe that as cleansing your mirror. If I can possibly help it, I have no wish to smudge that glass. So, I am determined to hold out against pills as long as possible.

Recently, that determination has been put to the test. I used to put myself to bed around 11 p.m., and get myself up around 6 a.m. Now that I can no longer get in and out of bed on my own, I have to have an attendant carer. I had expected, and dreaded, that I would be put to bed much earlier and be got up much later, which could have meant an extra two or three hours in bed. As the worst spasticity occurs first thing in the morning – which explains my early rising – those extra hours would be intolerable. Almost anything can trigger a vicious spasm from the tips of my toes through to the tips of the fingers of my left hand. My right is mercifully mostly exempt. When Fox was a young cat, he'd jump through the window and run straight up the bed towards me. Unless I bent my knees the moment I heard him jump through the window, I'd go into a vicious corpse spasm. The mere fact of having lain in almost the one position all night – I start on my right side and turn more or less onto my back after a few hours, where I stay until morning – produces repeated spasms. I've never timed them but they feel as if they are only a few minutes apart. The slightest movement, the slightest change in sensory signals, is also enough to trigger a painful spasm.

I needn't have worried. As it turns out, I am put to bed at the normal time and the carer arrives to get me up at 7 o'clock, so I have only one extra hour. One of her first chores is to give me some passive stretching, which helps to relax the spastic rigidity. I am sometimes so stiff and immovable that the carer has a terrible fight to persuade my leg to bend. I am still very uncomfortable from around 5 o'clock onwards, especially if it is hot or a nor'wester or both, and I have certainly been severely tempted to take anti-spasm. My carers, like most people, cannot understand my resistance to pills, so they have tried to persuade me to give in. In the meantime, however, I have decided to endure these two hours if that means I have a clear mind for the rest of the day.

More than six years ago, when I was still living in a house with stairs, I had asked the physio – we were distantly connected as she was Guy's second cousin and I had known her mother and grandmother slightly

– how other people managed when they were as bad as me.

She was categorical. 'They've given up,' she said. 'They're being looked after by their husband or wife, or they're in care. And, anyway, they're so zonked out on anti-spasm.'

'What do you mean?' I asked in surprise.

She explained. It was the first time I had known that it was, probably, only the spastic rigidity that was enabling me to stand at all. If I had given in and taken the dreaded pills and my muscles had become flaccid so that I could no longer support my own weight, I would have thought the MS had just taken another of its insidious turns for the worse. It would never have occurred to me to attribute my deterioration to the pills. And the doctor had not warned me. Instead he had blithely recommended them, warning me only about sleepiness. I was appalled. If the very pills you were taking could actually make you worse, what hope was there? I was tiptoeing through a minefield.

Maybe I was refusing to take anti-spasm but I was still dutifully swallowing my ulcer maintenance pill every evening. Then I had a visit from a medical student friend from Australia. He had been one of my tutorial students some 16 years before. He saw me take the pill and asked what it was for. I explained and told him my doctor's theory about anger. Pascall was enormously scornful. 'He's many years out of date,' he maintained. 'It's now known to be caused by a bacterium.'

I rang the doctor and tentatively mentioned the bacterium. Oh yes, he'd heard of it and agreed to write out a referral to the hospital. I went along, breakfastless, one morning, drank something, breathed into a bag and learnt that indeed I had the bacterium. Two weeks of antibiotics and a strong medication later and I was clear of the ulcer. That was four and a half years ago and, although I am still angry, the ulcer has not recurred.

I gained something else from Pascall's visit.

'I don't see,' he declared, 'why you can't visit friends in other parts of New Zealand. All you've got to do is tell them what equipment you need, they can hire it and there you are.'

At this, I became very distressed. 'You're treating me as if I were still the person I used to be,' I said pathetically.

He let the matter drop.

But that night while I was getting ready for bed, I thought about what he'd said and realised he was right. As my condition had deteriorated, I had narrowed my sights unnecessarily. I remembered a conversation when I had told a friend that my travelling days were over. She had said hers were too, because of her husband. I knew she meant because of her husband's health but the phrase wryly amused me and led to the poem: 'it's as if I spend my days/with a morose and unco-operative spouse'.

As a result of my conversation with Pascall, I organised a visit to Dunedin to my friend, Mary. She didn't need to hire any equipment, as her house was unusually accessible. There were no steps at the entrance so my electric wheelchair could just roll in; the lavatory was in the bathroom, so that was also manageable. The main difficulty was in my transfers from my wheelchair to an armchair. I become very un-comfortable if I'm forced to spend too much time in my wheelchair. I guess it's a circulation problem because my bottom goes to sleep. At home, I have had two chairs modified so that one arm can be lifted up to make it easier for me to effect my transfers. Without that raised arm, my transfers took much longer and involved a great deal of wriggling. A weekend visit was quite long enough. I could also survive two days without a shower, but wouldn't have liked to stay longer. I coped with the whole weekend, including the flight there and back, very well and gained much confidence in the process. I had enlarged my world.

But I didn't stop there. That conversation with Pascall and the visit to Mary led on to greater wonders. The following year in March a friend who suffers from a different neurological condition admitted she wished she could afford an attendant carer so that she could go to India.

'Why don't we share one and both go?' I heard myself say, something that would have been unthinkable six months earlier.

At the time, she agreed but, later, she had second thoughts. By then, I'd become quite excited about the thought of travelling again, even if India was likely to prove very difficult for someone in a wheelchair. I had even earmarked my current home help, Tessa, as a possible attendant carer. When the Indian idea fell through, I had convinced myself that I still wanted to go somewhere and that I wanted Tessa to go with me. Accordingly, Chile was the obvious choice. Tessa had had an AFS year there, knew Spanish and had loved the country. I put the idea to her. She agreed immediately.

'Don't you need time to think about it?' I asked.

'No,' she said.

'It will be like travelling with a middle-aged toddler,' I warned her. 'I may not indulge in tantrums and I'm a better conversationalist but you'll have to deal with the fact that my legs will often go in the opposite direction from the one you want them to go in. They seem to have a mind of their own.'

But she was unshaken. So, on 8 October 1995, we set off for a four-week stay. I had discovered we could get a LAN Chile air pass and visit many different places. Santiago was our base but we went as far north as Arica and as far south as Punta Arenas. We spent two days in Puerto Montt, another two in Tessa's AFS city, Chillan; we tracked down her host family who had moved to Concepción and stayed with them for a couple of days. A bus journey through the Andes to Mendoza in Argentina followed. It seemed a good idea, as we would be in the vicinity, to go to Easter Island, which is accessible only by LAN Chile, so we had a further two days there before returning to New Zealand via Tahiti. Altogether, it was a memorable time and we were justly proud of our achievement. I said Tessa knew some Spanish. I was wrong; she bubbled.

It is no slight undertaking, travelling when you are wheelchair-bound. Apart from Santiago, none of the airports had bridges so I had always to be carried up steps by officials, with Tessa frantically explaining that no, because of my spasticity, I couldn't just be carried up with a fireman's lift, that no, that was not where to pick up the wheelchair because those pieces came out in your hands. I had to accept, with a good grace, being manhandled. I had to smile and say, 'Gracias.' It was more difficult because I didn't know the language. It makes you feel very vulnerable being entirely dependent on someone with whom you can't communicate.

Tessa managed it all most staunchly. Initially, we had an arrangement that every few days we'd have a discussion about how we were coping, whether there was anything either of us was doing which the other found too difficult. But, after a couple of times, we discontinued this practice; it was not necessary.

On the strength of our successful Chilean adventure, we had a week last winter in Samoa, staying at Aggie Grey's. I found the heat and humidity very trying and was disappointed not to have a proper swim. Instead, I was dunked into the hotel pool once and into the sea twice and swilled around. Like a teabag, a friend suggested.

Last year, in October, I went to London with Pascall for a rushed, and all too brief fortnight. As a doctor, with a health clinic for

Aborigines, this was all he could spare. And at the moment, Tessa and I are anticipating our third overseas trip and are off shortly for a fortnight in the States, staying with friends in Oregon, then going back to San Francisco for a couple of days, with a final day in Los Angeles.

Chapter 11

During the first five and a half years that I lived in my present house, my major deteriorations came about as a result of accidents or my getting another illness. I have this theory that my body is providing all these troops to fight the MS. If something else goes wrong, I haven't got any reinforcements. I have to deploy some of the main army, leaving my flank exposed. Inevitably, this leads to a deterioration in the MS itself. There was one night when, after I had settled myself with my evening meal, I discovered I had forgotten to put the French dressing on my salad. I cursed but decided to get up again to rectify the problem. I was still able to walk a little. I can't have been paying close enough attention, because I fell and, this time, unlike most other times, I pulled a tendon in my left leg. I had a dreadful first night, having to ring out for help when I needed to get out of bed to go to the lavatory and again first thing in the morning. Indeed, for several nights, I had different people staying to help me in this way.

I gathered from the physio that, in normally active people, a torn tendon would take around six weeks to heal. Inevitably, it took longer than that for a woman with such limited mobility. I continued, stubbornly, doing yoga; only one of my, by now, very reduced repertoire of poses was really permanently affected by the injury but my walking became even more limited. In the end, gravity won out. I found I just couldn't lift my feet off the floor. All I could manage was the short walk from the scooter, parked outside the bedroom door, to the bed. This had become so unpleasant that it was almost a relief to give it up. I told one friend that I was no longer walking. She gave a long sigh of commiseration. I was feeling snarky.

'You weren't giving such a sigh,' I rebuked her unreasonably, 'when all I was doing was standing up, turning round and sliding backwards. That was all the walking I was managing.'

I don't remember that she made any reply. But then, what reply was possible?

My next injury was more serious. It was a day when I felt really right with the world. It was breakfast time and I was pouring boiling hot water from the jug into the teapot. To do that, I had to balance the lip of the jug on the edge of the pot. This particular morning, the jug slipped and I poured boiling hot water onto my feet. I don't wear shoes, only woollen socks, and as it took me far too long to remove them, in effect I was wearing boiling hot socks. Why I didn't go straight out and turn the garden tap on my feet, I really don't know. I'd certainly do that if I happened to burn myself again. Instead, I gave myself third-degree burns on both feet. They blistered; they were red and swollen. The pain was severe and caused frequent spasms, when I'd suddenly jerk backwards. Driving a car in such circumstances was obviously out of the question, so until the pain, and the jerks, subsided, I had to get wheelchair taxis to the university.

After I had removed my socks, I called a friend and then the doctor's surgery. My doctor came, with his nurse, both very concerned; he wanted to put me into hospital. I refused.

'I can't go into hospital,' I insisted. 'My Fox-pussy's got a broken jaw.'

Luckily, the doctor had no jurisdiction and couldn't force me to go. I offered a more cogent objection.

'They'll put me in a burns ward where they'll know nothing about MS. Or they'll put me in an MS ward where they'll know nothing about burns and I'll be fighting every inch of the way.'

He had, perforce, to concur. It was only later that I was told I stood more chance of getting an infection in hospital than I did at home. Apparently, I'm used to the bugs at home and I would have less resistance to new ones in the hospital.

So, I stayed at home with nurses coming, at first, twice a day to dress the burns. Then I was promoted to once a day, then twice a week until finally I was pronounced healed. The right foot took longer to mend than the left because I managed to get the left sock off first, and even now, three years later, the skin on the right foot can look more like plastic than actual skin.

I took a tranquilliser so that I could sleep on the first night and painkillers for the first few days. But these had no effect on the actual pain; they just altered my perception of it. As I can do that myself, I stopped taking them. The unexpected, jerking spasms stopped after a couple of weeks, so that I could go back to driving. Showering was impossible unless I had someone here to put my feet in plastic bags; it wouldn't have been a good idea for me to sit in wet, soggy bandages all day.

I burnt my feet the day before the first tutorials of the year. The students in my classes had a good introduction to me as I had to request a lot of help. I always sit with my feet stretched out on a stool to ease the spasticity and improve my circulation. For up to 10 minutes, I have the left leg stretched out straight and the right one on the edge of the stool with the knee bent out to the right; then I reverse the position by pulling on my socks, the only way I can move my legs. This reduces my body's predilection for foetal spasticity. It stops my knees being locked permanently in a bent position. So that I can change my position, I wear knee-high pure wool socks – a trace of synthetic and my hand slips as I pull. This is a nuisance as it means that I have to wear wool, even in the heat of summer. When I had massive bandages on my feet, I couldn't wear socks, and so I couldn't lift my feet up on to the stool in the first place, nor change their position once they were there. I, therefore, had to ask students I'd never met before to help me. Nothing like throwing them in the deep end!

It was even worse during the long hours I was on my own. I must change the position of my legs at regular intervals. Otherwise, I have a vicious spastic reaction. It is one of the prices I pay for not taking anti-spasm. In addition, I needed to yank on my socks to get the feet up on the bed so that I could do yoga. A friend made me a stirrup arrangement that I could slip over my foot. I could then lift or pull the foot, whichever was needed. It wasn't easy but, at least, it was possible.

But I lost an important yoga pose and my twice daily exercycling stint. These, particularly the latter, had been strengthening and exercising my leg muscles. Without them, my muscles weakened to the point where I could no longer take my weight. The standing and stretching I had done in the past, and had to apologise to students about, had long become a taking of my weight on my arms so that my bottom would rise just a little off the seat. This was especially useful for putting my bathing costume on. After I'd burnt my feet, I found that I could no longer lift my bottom. I really missed this, as it had been a way of ensuring that my bottom didn't go to sleep. Sitting all day as I do, I can get very uncomfortable.

One of the major difficulties of managing on my own was that, when I put myself to bed, I couldn't get myself far enough into it. I have a three-quarter bed, which would give me plenty of room, if only I was able to take advantage of it. But I could sit only far enough into the bed for my knees to be right on the edge and my feet on the floor. Any further in, and my legs would have been sticking straight out in front of me. When I lifted my legs onto the bed, therefore, they were very close to the edge. And even if I came up on my elbow and managed to push them further into the bed, my right hip and buttock were still as close to the edge as ever. This had two dire consequences.

I'd wake in the early hours of the morning and find both feet out of the bed. Because the blood had been pooling in them, the feet looked dreadful: purple and angry. The burn scars looked particularly unpleasant. But, worse, because the legs had been out of the bed for goodness knows how long, they had become heavy and inert, which made it very difficult for me to lift them back into bed. Often, once I had managed to sit up, it would take 10 minutes to get the legs, by this time frozen, back into the bed. I managed to remain philosophical about this, when it happened about once a month, even though it was really unpleasant on a cold, frosty mid-winter night.

But in 1998, we had a particularly hot summer with numerous nor'westers. Far from the legs coming out of the bed only once a month, they started coming out three, or even four, times a night. I was utterly exhausted. Each time they came out, it would take me 15-20 minutes to get them back into bed, another 10 minutes or more to get back to sleep, and blow me down, an hour or so later, they'd be out again. With each time they came out, it was harder to get them as far back into the bed as I could manage the first time. This meant that each time the legs came out, the more likely it was that they'd come out again.

I was getting really desperate. I asked everyone I could think of if they could come up with a solution, but nobody could find any way out of the problem. I was told, as I had been told so many times before, that when people were as bad as me, they didn't try to manage on their own, so this problem had never been addressed before. I thought this was a stupid avoidance. If I had still been married to Guy, they seemed to be saying, it would be fine for me to wake him three or four times a night – although I suppose he'd have been able to ensure my legs were far enough into the bed in the first place, that they wouldn't have been coming out in this disagreeable manner. In desperation, I gave the problem some more thought. If the sheet and duvet were to be tucked in, I wouldn't be able to get my legs out of the bed at all. I seemed to be stuck at an impasse. It looked as if I was going to be forced to endure such unpleasant interrupted nights indefinitely, or at least while I was still putting myself to bed.

Then it occurred to me to try raising the mattress slightly at the point where my feet were coming out. I had to be careful how much it was raised: too much would undoubtedly keep the feet in at night, but would make it too difficult for me to get them out in the morning. That, after all, was hard enough to manage. Visualise it. I am reclining on my right elbow. I can hook my left hand round my right knee and yank. This brings the right leg out. The left poses more of a problem. It is often lying along the bed, stretched straight out. A full bladder is likely to produce this problem with the left leg. It's not only straight, it's ramrod straight, which makes it very heavy and unpliable. Yet, until I can get the knee to bend a little, I can get no purchase on the leg. I am reduced to poking desperately behind the knee with the curved end of a walking stick until I can persuade the knee to bend. Then I can try pulling at the calf muscle to persuade the leg out of the bed. This is hard enough without making the leg slide uphill. So, if the mattress were to be raised, it had to be just enough and no more. What was needed, I found, was a cushion. I could accommodate the extra difficulty this added to my getting out of bed because my feet went back to coming out only once a month.

Both feet out was one difficulty. Another was that I'd wake and find my left leg had spasmed itself out across the right leg. Sometimes it was possible, without actually sitting up, to grab hold of it and force it back into the bed beyond the right one. Mostly, however, I had to struggle to sit up, and I mean struggle. Next I would bring the wheelchair alongside the bed until I could get the offending foot onto the footplate. I also needed to bring the right foot out of the bed, but it was anchored too firmly by the weight of the left leg across it. Fortunately, my wheelchair can be raised and lowered. When I raised it, of course, the left leg was raised too, which took some of the weight off the other leg. By judicious tugging, I could eventually get the right foot out so that I could then lower it to the floor. This had to be negotiated very carefully, or I'd bang the foot down hard against the wheelchair. It's not just that that would hurt; any unexpected, especially painful sensory signal can cause me to jerk uncontrollably backward, as I had done when I burnt my feet. So, I had to be especially careful. Now I had both feet down, it was just a case of once more moving the wheelchair down towards the foot of the bed and once more struggling to get my legs back into the bed. All these manoeuvrings had to be executed by a person without balance. At any time, there was the risk that I'd tip sideways or backwards and be unable to reach the phone to ring for help. If I remembered, before I'd begin the whole undertaking, I'd place the cordless phone on the bed beside me.

I often, in these years, wished I had four hands. At my request, an occupational therapist brought a gadget for me to try which was supposed to make lifting the legs easier. It wasn't free-standing, so I had to hold it with one hand. If I'm not wearing socks, which, of course I'm not when I'm about to get into bed, I need two hands to lift my leg even the littlest bit off the ground. I'm perched on the edge of the bed and have to hold onto the bed rail to stop me tipping sideways. Altogether, that makes four hands. I returned the lifting gadget to the therapist.

While I was endeavouring to sort out what to do about my feet falling out of bed, an occupational therapist came to watch my getting into bed techniques. I heaved the left leg up onto the bed, grabbed the right with both hands and simultaneously, because of my bad balance, threw myself back, bringing my right leg up with me. She, obviously, found this too strenuous and offered me a hospital bed that could be electronically tilted.

I looked at her in amazement. 'What does it matter if I get tired just as I am about to get into bed?' I asked her. 'I have to use my body, don't I?'

She looked dumbfounded.

Chapter 12

In 1996, one of the nurses who came to dress my burnt feet was a continence adviser. She found it extraordinary that, despite the fact that my walk had completely disappeared, I still had bladder control. That was over three years ago and I am still catheterised only when I am travelling. Fortunately, I have suffered bladder infections only when I am catheterised. I attribute my successful bladder control to a book I read about MS ages ago when I was in Melbourne. The female writer indicated that one of the reasons women are more prone to bladder infections than men, is that they don't empty their bladders properly. She recommended leaning forward when you think you've finished, to put slight pressure on the bladder. I tried it and she was right. Although I was convinced I had emptied my bladder completely, there was always about a tablespoon of urine left. So I made the leaning forward part of my routine.

As the MS has progressed I have had more and more bladder retention. So, in addition to leaning forward at the end of peeing, I have taken to kneading my bladder as if I were making bread. Recently, I have introduced yet another strategy. I recognised that I needed to provide a sensory signal to the urethra; accordingly, I touch it gently with the handle of an old toothbrush, then I lean forward. I find such stimulus encourages the bladder to empty properly which reduces the risk of infection. It also means I am retaining control. Mindful of the tendency of MS to make the body forget skills, when I have a catheter, I always have one with a valve. I can then open it when I need to pee, and close it off the rest of the time. Thus, when the catheter is finally removed, I am back to what, for me, is normal.

I remember asking the continence nurse why other people didn't practise what I have heard described as 'toilet acrobatics'. She indicated they couldn't be bothered. I realise that, if I were catheterised, I could visit friends – it's not just access to their houses but to their lavatories which is a problem – and I would need fewer carers, but I loathe the intrusiveness. And, as I will explain shortly, the supra-pubic one I briefly tried before I went to London was no better.

Some years ago my occupational therapist suggested permanent catheterisation and looked very surprised when I gave a firm 'No!' I wondered whether, given that I might just as well need a lavatory because of a bowel movement, she would next suggest I have a colostomy so that I wouldn't ever need a lavatory at all. To do her justice, however, she was also concerned because I was having difficulty, in the afternoons, my worst time of day, with my standing transfers off the lavatory. I would make several attempts to stand up, but to no avail. I'd sometimes end up shouting at my recalcitrant body, 'I'm only trying to stand up. I'm not trying to climb Mount Everest.' And I'd burst into tears. That usually worked, although I don't know why. Obviously, this situation couldn't last indefinitely. The day would come when I just wouldn't stand up at all. The problem was solved in the end by raising the lavatory an inch or so. In the light of the look of surprise on the occupational therapist's face when I turned down her catheter suggestion, I subsequently asked the physio whether other people did what they were told.

'They don't know their own minds the way you do,' she replied.

I later discussed the occupational therapist's suggestion with various medical people who all agreed I was far too young to be permanently catheterised unless it were strictly necessary, so I was glad I had been so bloody-minded.

As a result of the struggle to get myself into bed, I learnt something else about how the body functions. For example, I would need to lift one leg across the other. In this way, one foot came off the floor, which made it easier to get my sock off. Some nights, it lifted on the first try. Others, I was still trying after four or five attempts. I discovered that if I said, 'Lift, damn you!', my foot mostly took no notice. But, if I said, 'Please lift, because until you do, I can't get my sock off and until my sock is off, I can't get into bed. And I'm tired and really want to get to sleep', then it lifted on the next try. I was told I was accessing a different part of my brain. I wish I'd known this when I was still attempting the stairs. I might have gone on walking longer, even if I were in danger of being locked up for talking to myself. The habit of explaining things to my body spread, until I have even caught myself explaining to the tin-opener why I wanted it to work, because the cats were hungry, wanted their dinner and there'd be a riot if I didn't feed them soon.

For many years now, I have started the day with yoga breathing. I don't think I should glorify what I do by calling it *Pranyama*. My reasons for doing this yoga breathing are two-fold. First, it's obviously good for me, when I am otherwise so sedentary, to extend my breathing capacity. Although MS is not a killer, pneumonia is one of the secondary risks. My other reason is that we breathe in accordance with our emotional state. Changing our breathing means we also change our emotional state. I had a friend, for instance, with ankylosing spondylitis, which causes stiffening and immobility of the joints; I gave her some breathing instruction. But, because of the induced rigidity of her rib cage, her breathing capacity was severely limited. Indeed, she thought that breathing in and out to the count of two each time meant that she was breathing deeply. Her normal breathing was one second in and one second out – panic breathing. No wonder she was depressed. I can manage much longer cycles than two seconds in and out. In fact, whenever a doctor tells me to breathe deeply, I am usually only halfway through when I am expected to stop.

'You don't want me to breathe deeply,' I accuse the doctor, 'you want me to breathe quickly.'

My morning routine has me working up to a 12-second in and out, with retention on every third breath. I do this each day, but I'll also do it at other times if I feel I need to calm myself down. We're all familiar with the injunction to take a deep breath, if we're feeling hot and bothered. Well, I can vouch for its efficacy.

Yoga always instructs you to do each movement on an out breath. When I'm having particular trouble with a familiar movement, changing the position of my feet on my stool perhaps, I notice my breathing, take one or two deep breaths, then try again on an out breath. I'm usually successful with this technique.

For several years after I came out of remission, I had been seeing an acupuncturist. Just before I shifted in 1993, he said that I lived on the edge. And certainly, people who came to assess me from time to time were always amazed that I was managing without attendant carers to get me up, give me a shower and put me to bed.

Showering was the first to go. Although I hadn't had an emergency where I couldn't manage to slide on or off the shower stool, something in me said 'Enough!' The risks I was running just became too much for me to handle, and I arranged for someone to come in and help me. Sadly, that meant a shower on only three days and a lick and a promise on the other four.

Before I had set this assistance in place, I mentioned to a counsellor that I was panicking about having a shower.

'Oh, are you afraid of the water?' she asked.

'No,' I corrected her. 'I'm afraid I'm not going to be able to get on and off the shower stool.'

She had the grace to look sheepish. But her misinterpretation of my remark highlighted for me a problem I had often encountered: the tendency of others to take metaphorically something I meant literally. So, I'd say, 'I'm off balance', and some people would assume I was having trouble with my inner ear. But you'd be surprised at those who assumed that I was psychologically off balance, that my mind was disturbed in some way. I think this has something to do with the bizarre quality of neurological symptoms. People are less comfortable with them so they choose to interpret what I say within more familiar paradigms.

So, I now had help with my shower and, not long after, I had to compromise my independence again and acquire the security alarm. As you can see, I was even more precariously on the edge. Then I fell over, and although it was, initially, a very slight deterioration, I never managed to scramble back up. I think that if I hadn't gone to London in 1999 with my friend, Pascall, I might have held on a bit longer. But not much.

I don't want to deny the reality of my changed condition but I see now that it's not so much that the MS has worsened, as that my ability to manage it has lessened.

Going to London brought about one such change. Having the wheelchair seat recovered without making sure the new seat had a slippery surface was another. The non-slip surface created a vacuum between me and the seat so that I frequently stuck solid. The struggle to release myself put an enormous strain on my already weak left arm. There were even times when I was stuck so fast that I had to ring for help. As well, I developed a callus on my right buttock, which made sliding transfers very painful. The London trip compounded my difficulties. Obviously I had to be catheterised again. I was most reluctant, but had no choice. Although I had survived the Samoan holiday without infection, I had had a massive bladder infection after I returned from Chile. In the hopes that my risk of infection would be minimised, it was decided, although it was for so short a time, that I should have a supra-pubic catheter instead of a urethral one.

It seemed as if I deteriorated immediately. I don't know whether it was that my body rejected this invasion of its territory or whether I developed an infection straight away, but even by the time the taxi had delivered me home from the hospital I was feeling negative effects. I intended sitting out in the garden until lunchtime. As I left the back door open in such circumstances, I needed to put the cats' plates away in a drawer so that none of the other cats that prowled the garden could come and steal the remains of their breakfast. After all the years of yoga, I bend from the hips, so I bent down but could not straighten up again. It took me about 10 minutes of struggling before I was upright once more and, all that time, I was worrying whether I could reach either the security medallion or the cellphone that sits on the footplate of the wheelchair.

That was the start of a slow decline. I had to arrange for friends to stay the night to help me get into bed and up again in the morning. It signalled the total loss of my independence.

With a supra-pubic catheter, you are supposed to be able to pee normally. On two of the six days before I had this catheter removed, I could, on one or two occasions, pee a little. By then, I definitely had an infection and so was on antibiotics. On the morning of my departure for Australia, I had a urethral catheter inserted, some four days after I had had the other removed. So I set off for my grand British tour, already depleted of energy. I was decidedly off colour just when I needed all my emotional reserves to cope with the exigencies of the trip and the nostalgic impact of returning, after two and a half decades, to my home of 10 years.

I sailed through the fortnight with flying colours, buoyed up, I imagine, by the intellectual stimulus and exhilaration of being back in London. We went to three concerts and three plays; I caught up with various friends from the past; I was taken back to the street where I used to live, but it had gone so upmarket it was hardly recognisable. I expected to be haunted by a small boy in a blue duffle-coat. What I hadn't expected was to feel so completely that I had come home.

The journey back to New Zealand was appallingly difficult, despite my taking a tranquilliser so that I could sleep for some of the time. It is a long, hard undertaking for anyone, flying straight from London to Melbourne. When you can't stand up or change your position at all, it is far worse. The spasticity in my legs was atrocious, and continued to be so for several days after my return. I had to take a tranquilliser for several nights before I weaned myself off them as I didn't want to become too dependent. While we were away, Pascall had regularly performed a sort of litmus paper test on my urine and this revealed that I had a persistent low-level bladder infection. He treated this with antibiotics. The infection was still there on my return so I had to swallow even more pills. At least at home, I could also eat acidopholous yoghurt to neutralise any of the harmful effects of the antibiotics.

Despite this, I returned home riding high emotionally, after all I had achieved. I had the richest of memories. Okay, I was still fragile, but it had taken me a week to get myself right after the week in Samoa. But this was a longer time away; I had jet lag and a bladder infection, so it would take me longer to regain my independence. It took me a while to realise that I would never regain it. After so many years of balancing so precariously, I had fallen over the edge.

A friend used to say that if I was half an inch out, I couldn't manage. Now I was permanently that half an inch out and, indeed, I couldn't manage. The major problem was my sliding transfers. I assumed when I came back from England that I could do them as I used to do. With difficulty and perseverance, I transferred from my armchair to the wheelchair and from there to the lavatory. It was while getting off the lavatory that I ended up in a reef knot on the floor with the phone off the hook and nobody responding when I pressed the medallion round my neck. After this alarming episode, I struggled on for several days, hoping that everything would come right but it became increasingly obvious that I was always going to need help with the transfers. Accordingly, regular care was set in place. An army of carers entered my life; I had been colonised.

During the first week of care, I thought I'd go out of my mind. The carers occupy over 40 hours of the week: it's as if I have a full-time job. Each carer, and there were many, had to be taught what to do. I can't cope with people coming into my house as strangers; when I was a relieving teacher, I used to waste enormous amounts of energy trying to establish genuine contact and rapport with students I would never see again. So, in addition to having to explain all the different techniques the carers needed to assimilate in order to assist me, I wore myself out trying to connect with a whole range of people whose life experiences and interests were very different from mine. When you consider the number of hours I was spending in the company of my carers, you will begin to understand the difficulties I was facing. I don't, after all, spend that much time with my closest friends. I have made several friends among the members of the choir I have been in for 12 years. If nothing else, we have in common our love of singing and of the particular music we sing. What the carers and I had in common, initially, was the fact that my body doesn't work properly. That's not exactly an exhilarating topic. We needed to establish something else we could share.

My university education and work have meant that I know a fairly narrow cross-section of society and most of my friends have similar connections. Unlike my Paul who, when he was living in a commune in Australia, had to conceal his sophisticated knowledge of European art, I am unable to keep a low profile and say, 'Oh yeah, gidday.' Now, suddenly, I not only had to create relationships with a wider array of people but I had to accept from them, with a smile, the gross violations of privacy that come with being disabled. Now, it is easier because, yes, I have established contact, which has made my carers into real people and I no longer suffer such fastidious recoil. But, in the beginning, this need to turn my carers into real people was another drain on my already shaky energy.

Chapter 13

It is only now that I realise the very great emotional adjustment I have had to make. I have lost privacy, freedom, independence; I have had to accept an invasion of my house; and I have had to fully acknowledge my disability for the first time, with all the horror and disbelief that this has involved. And, in addition, I have to be grateful. However much I am mourning the loss of being able to get myself in and out of bed, I have to pretend that this is fine by me. I have to be pleasant, polite and civilised while I have a suppository inserted or my creases are examined to make sure that I am not running the risk of developing a rash. I have to accept being treated very much as a helpless child while, at the same time, remaining an adult. I have, simultaneously, to surrender power and to maintain it.

I'm glad to recall that, although I had become so helpless and dependent, I didn't retreat into a state of passivity. I devised, almost immediately, ways of enhancing my life. If I was going to be stranded in my bed an hour or so longer in the morning, I needed something better than the portable radio I had bought in 1980 for my parents' 50th wedding anniversary. I had quite a collection of CDs which I hadn't been listening to; a radio/CD player with a remote control would solve both those problems.

It was now, too, that after 20 years, I acquired a television and video. I had hired one for the young friend who had house sat while I was in England. Another friend had lent me various videos. After I'd been back only a few days, and was feeling decidedly lacklustre, I had watched Ian McKellen's stunning version of *Richard III*. I recognised that such videos could provide me with much-missed intellectual stimulus.

Then I worked out that, if I could no longer get myself onto my wheelchair whenever I wanted, I was going to be mostly in the same room. Attractive as it is, I knew I needed changes of scene. I have a large house with other rooms. One, a delightful sunroom, was too full of plants. A shelf and a few more hooks so the plants could be hung solved that problem. I now spend many afternoons in a different room with a completely changed outlook.

There was another room I hardly ever used. When I first shifted, I was in it quite often because it contains the piano, and, since it was large, I could teach yoga in it. But, first of all, my piano playing went and the yoga class shrank to two people, whom I could accommodate in my sitting room. The big room, as I imaginatively call it, is exactly that: big. You can see that it has been enlarged. It looks out across the park and faces south and west. With a high stud as well, it is expensive to heat. It had an open fire, which I never used, so I decided to get a gas heater installed in the fireplace in order to spend time in there. My sitting room has a wood burner but I can no longer manage to put fuel on it myself, so I have taken to having it lit only when I am having an evening visitor. The rest of the time I have an electric heater with a thermostat. Gas is, obviously, more expensive because it is a large heater which I'm not able to turn on and off, but it is very pleasant to be able to have a change of venue.

All these enhancements were expensive and I could never have managed if my uncle and godmother had not been most generous. They were wealthy, had no children and were very good to all their nieces and nephews. As goddaughter, I was in a special category, and, as a little girl, I had had golden ringlets. Without their money, I wouldn't have been able to buy this house or even contemplate my overseas trips.

When my friends come to see me now, I am sitting in my chair, just as I was when I was still maintaining my independence. The fact that I am losing function in my left arm and hand, which means that my hand looks slightly puffy and unused, or that it is clawing with the thumb tightly squeezed by the fingers and I cannot open the fingers out, is not, after all, very conspicuous. As it happens, I don't look any more or less disabled than I did this time last year. And I am very assertive and articulate. I present myself, quite deliberately, in a positive fashion. My clown's mask is firmly in place. If you take all this into account, then it's no wonder that people assume I am less disabled than is the case. It would almost be true to say that I invite such a misconception. That was okay when I was still independent. I'm finding it less palatable now that I am so needy.

One of the problems is that MS is chronic. There's no drama in such a condition. It's not sensational. It's rather boring. It won't go away. Like the weather, it's here to stay. I remember how newsworthy it was when I came out of remission. There was a sharp difference between my walking quite normally and my struggling along on sticks. Now, the changes, world-shattering as they are for me, don't have the same impact.

And, to tell the truth, I don't really know how friends react to my disability. A couple have indicated they feel somewhat guilty because they are all right and I am not. This makes me anxious that such feelings of guilt may cause them to want to avoid me. Another friend has indicated that, when I tell her how it is for me, and I certainly don't do so all that often, it makes her feel helpless. I believe her. I remember an exchange of many years ago, when I was still managing to walk a short distance. I had been having a bad day. When she rang, I blurted out, 'I can't walk.'

'I can't do anything about that,' she replied, with real pain in her voice.

I should have said, 'Yes, you can let me talk about it.' But I didn't and her sad and regretful helplessness effectively silenced me.

More recently, when she has acknowledged that she feels helpless, I have tried to explain that there are two aspects of having MS: there's the coping with the actual physical difficulties and there's the loneliness that comes from feeling that this is how it is and nobody understands. Letting me talk occasionally helps to reduce that feeling of isolation. But I remember only too well the pain of watching Paul suffer and not being able to do anything except love him and be there, with and for him. I so wanted to be able to kiss the sore spot to make it better. So, I understand how it is for others, even while I am battling my feelings of isolation.

The whole time that I was struggling to come to terms with the changes in my physical condition and the fear as to what the future would hold, I still had to deal with the army of carers. It took some time before I had a regular number. Certainly, a great many tried me out but, for various reasons, were not suitable. My transfers from wheelchair to bed or armchair are effected by putting a sliding board under me, making sure there is skirt or nightie between me and the board, and then pulling the skirt. In this way, I slide onto the wheelchair or chair. But I cannot be slid in this way onto the shower stool or lavatory. There, I have to be lifted. I have a hoist but most of my present carers prefer not to use it. At the beginning, when I was only a few weeks away from sliding on and off the lavatory without needing help and was still managing half of that movement myself, I was loath to accept the undoubted fact that I needed a hoist. So I didn't encourage the carers to use it. In fact, I actively discouraged them; the hoist remained in a spare room with the door closed.

Although I had, by now, a number of regular carers, there were still various slots where the organising agency had difficulty in providing me with enough helpers. This was partly due to the number of hours of care I required each day, since I am not catheterised. The other reason was that I still expected carers to lift me on and off the lavatory. Various people found the lifting beyond them. It was no use telling them they'd find it would get easier if they were willing to persevere. They weren't willing, and that was all there was to it. You will gather that I was being totally unreasonable and discounting their fully justified fears.

Lately, I have shifted ground and, instead of living in an egocentric bubble, where my needs were the only ones that counted and I ignored the difficulties and risks my carers were undergoing on my behalf, I am offering the hoist to all of them. So far, they have all refused it, for which I am very grateful, but now that is their decision, not mine.

I realise that I am making it sound as if the hoist will solve all my problems. After all, I have never used one myself and, therefore, do not know how difficult it is. But I have been given to understand that using a hoist is not just a rigmarole; it is heavier work than I'd supposed. I mean, if I'm hoisted off my present chair, it's not likely that I will be positioned on the wheelchair so that I can drive myself into the bathroom only to have to be hoisted again onto the lavatory. I'll be dragged, still on the hoist, into the bathroom. Hoists are for lifting. They don't move easily with a dead weight swinging. Managing a hoist, therefore, requires a different kind of strength and skill than lifting me. It still demands a great deal of my carers.

Anyway, I really had no notion what a trial I was being, at this time, to the co-ordinator for my area, until she dropped a bombshell on me. She asked whether she could come and see me. The date was 30 March, a few days before Easter. At this meeting, I was told that, as of 6 April, they were withdrawing their services because it was proving too difficult to provide adequate carers. It was suggested I turn to one of the other two care-providing agencies in Christchurch.

I had already rejected the idea of one of these agencies since they weren't flexible; you had to have whoever they sent you and couldn't provide any helpers of your own choosing. Over the years, I had always preferred to find my own home helps. I would get a young person through Student Job Search; much less set in their ways, students were easier to train. They didn't try and impose their ways on me. The agency I had chosen had, somewhat reluctantly, allowed my student helpers to register with them on a casual basis. If, now, I turned to another agency, I would lose that advantage. And, when I remembered the difficulty I had had breaking in new carers, my heart sank. There was no way I wanted to go through that again.

I set myself to negotiate with the co-ordinator. That meant, however angry I was at being treated in what I felt was a cavalier manner, I must conceal it and respond as reasonably as I could. I did say mildly that I thought I was being given very short notice. She seemed to think a week, which included Easter, was quite sufficient. I only hinted at the fact that I had been advised to contact the *Holmes Show*. I rather think I was expected to roll over and play dead. Instead, I appealed to be allowed to keep the carers from the agency who had regular slots with me and assured her I would take up the slack and find other carers.

I mooted the idea of getting my own funding. A Christchurch woman had recently succeeded in taking over her own funding arrangements. I had met her and she had found that this approach worked very well. She could choose who she wanted to work for her, could pay them more and, most importantly, it restored to her some sense of being in control of her own life. The suggestion that I might follow her example was greeted very half-heartedly. The rest of my proposition was given approval. I was to retain the services of all those who had been coming to me on and off for several months, I was relaxed and comfortable with them and we had established a routine. I had less explaining to do. Indeed, when I remind one of my carers that I want her to do something, she grumbles that I am becoming boringly repetitive, not to say, obsessional. But not everyone remembers as well as she does.

These carers, with an occasional helping-out visit from another person, provided about two-thirds of the care I needed. I had spoken most confidently about taking up the slack: now I had to put my words into practice. At first, I called mainly on previous home helps; then I acquired another student and a qualified nurse. I am now at the stage where there are only a few slots in the week where I have no regular helpers and I even, to a certain extent, have back-ups. It's rather like not relying on my hard disk but having a second copy on floppy.

One of the problems I have had is that my carers are often more conventional than me; they would call it more tidy. Like my mother, they fail to understand my insouciance about dust, unironed clothes or the fact that my hair looks like a bird's nest – I have an almost permanent toddler tangle at the back because, in bed, I lie either on my right side or my back and can't turn over. Also I can't easily brush or comb it out. I once embarrassed one of the carers when she, very kindly, came swimming with me. She objected to walking beside me on the way to the pool because I was still in my, not very obvious, tartan nightie – after all, why should I put clothes on, only to have to take them off again? – and I refused to let her tidy my hair because I was about to get it wet through.

At the beginning, until I protested, the carers were all set to reorganise both me and my house. At first, I tolerated it, but, in the end, I called a halt. 'Let me live my own life,' I declared.

It helps that I am so assertive. I can well imagine someone passively accepting the interference of his or her carers, while secretly resenting it. It's important that there should be an ease, a relaxed acceptance between carers and the person they are helping; buried resentment would be counter-productive.

In this new and difficult enterprise of getting to know all these various people, I have found humour a great help. Rachael, whom I got through Student Job Search, told me that one of her fellow students used to work for a young paraplegic woman who had been paralysed since her mid-teens. If anything went wrong, this woman would blame her helper, claiming that she didn't like her and was deliberately hurting her. I was amazed but, when I asked my other carers, they indicated they'd met with the same irrational reception.

So Rachael and I decided to turn this into a game. She was pulling me forward on the wheelchair by holding me under the thighs.

'You pulled one of the hairs on my leg,' I pointed out. 'That's not very delicate.'

'It's because I don't like you,' she insisted smugly.

And we'd giggle together.

Another game relates to my accidentally running over a carer's feet with my wheelchair. It's quite unintentional. But, by the same token, so is their standing on my toes. 'Oh good!' I say. 'Now I can run you over.' It keeps us good-humoured and there is no blame.

Then there was one night when I was being helped into bed and the sliding board had slipped on my satin under-sheet, so that it had jammed itself with the sharp edge under my thigh. I was too near the edge of the bed for it to be pulled out frontwards. That would risk my falling onto the floor. I was going to have to be slid further onto the bed first, which would inevitably hurt.

'What say I shriek first,' I suggested. 'You know, like *Alice Through the Looking Glass*, where you're put in prison first and then can commit your crime.'

It worked. I shrieked, she pulled and it seemed less painful than it might otherwise have done. We were most amused.

The young friend who has been coming to help me out for over six years, and who is particularly important because she assists me with a couple of yoga poses I can no longer manage on my own, has said it helps that, when things go wrong, instead of my throwing a tantrum, I'm likely to collapse in a fit of giggles. I don't know where such a reaction comes from, but it certainly is the case that, when I end up in a totally unsuitable position, provided it doesn't hurt, I'll most probably get the giggles.

I've also had to learn to be patient. When I was thanking Tessa for being so gentle with me when we were in Chile, she said my being so patient helped. I mentioned to Guy once that I'd had to acquire patience, knowing that he, of all people, would have been aware that it didn't come naturally to me. 'You will have gone about acquiring it with your usual fierce intent,' he suggested.

It also seems most important to me that, no matter how grouchy I'm feeling, I treat my carers with courtesy and respect. They are people with their own needs. I've asked several of them what really irks them about their clients. They like to feel valued, like to feel the work they do is appreciated. Just because I'd rather they didn't have to do it is no reason for me to be disagreeable.

One of the most difficult aspects for both MS sufferers and their carers is the confusion that results from damage to the sensory nerves. We experience the world through sight, hearing, smell, touch and taste and if any of the signals are distorted, it is hard for us to recognise that we are the ones who have the world wrong.

I have very damaged sensory nerves and I have located three areas where this can cause difficulty. In the first place, MS sufferers, who, like me, have an exaggerated response, are the original princess with the pea under the mattress. I interpret the smallest tuck or fold of my skirt or nightdress as a large clump of material. I squirm and wriggle as if something really bulky is digging into me. I explain to the carer that I'm not comfortable because, even though she has already smoothed it out, my clothing is, to me, still all bunched up. I have to explain to my body that, while it feels uncomfortable, it has got it wrong. It is lying on a perfectly smooth surface.

If you add such an exaggerated response to the fact that my body doesn't know where it is in space, you get other problems. I asked a carer the other night, when she had just got me into bed, to straighten my left leg. It felt, to me, as if the knee was bent quite considerably. 'It is straight,' she said in surprise.

This relates to the second problem: my nerves don't turn off quickly enough. I continue to receive the message for a minute or more after it is no longer appropriate. The easiest example of this is that, for some time after I have taken off my rings before going to bed, I still can feel them on my fingers. Last night, the feeling was so strong, that, despite the fact that I could distinctly remember taking them off, I had to look at my fingers just to make sure.

Then again, I notice the difficulty with my legs. Part of my yoga practice each day is a pose where I sit with one leg stretched straight out in front of me, the other bent so the sole of the foot nestles against the opposite thigh and I lie along the straight leg. I hold the pose for a quarter of an hour. The problem occurs when I need to change the pose. When the bent leg is straightened, it takes a minute at the very least for it to register that it is now straight. It retains the memory of its bentness. I have to instruct the carer who is helping me with my yoga poses to lean gently on the knee until it starts remembering that it is straight.

Once, way back when I was still walking, I had been sitting with my legs crossed under me. The phone rang and I stood up to go and answer it. The trouble was that as far as my legs were concerned, they were still crossed. They crumpled under me and I fell.

This delayed reaction poses other problems: if a carer moves me too vigorously, my body cannot adjust in time. Unless I am moved gently, my body spasms and jerks in protest. It can sound as if I'm just nit-picking when I ask a carer to move me more slowly and carefully. But with my lack of proprioceptive awareness, my unstable balance, my body cannot process abrupt movements and changes of position. As you would imagine, this can create tension between me and carers if they are feeling pressured in other ways. Then I can sense their impatience and frustration. There was one, at the beginning, who had no patience at all for my repeated requests to position my legs in a particular way before attempting to move me. I wanted to scream at her, 'You silly bitch, will you listen to what I'm telling you. After nearly 30 years of yoga, I know my body and its capabilities better than you.' But I didn't, because it wouldn't have been appropriate. After sessions with this particular carer, I used to feel as if all my energy had been leached out of me. Luckily, before something drastic could go wrong, there was a minor problem, which led to her not coming again.

There was one other carer I couldn't cope with. I would say her reasons for choosing to be a carer were pathological; she needed to be needed. To achieve this end, she had to reduce me to a state of total helplessness. In transactional analysis terms, she had adopted the role of rescuer. This meant that, whether I wanted it or not, I was cast in the role of victim. I was so angry and frustrated that, in no time at all, I was playing out the role of persecutor. Fortunately, before we could do one another psychological damage, she chose to leave. She found me too much. I don't know whether she realised how relieved I would be. The episode with this woman came early on in my experience of caregivers. I hope I'd handle the whole situation more diplomatically now.

My mind works very quickly, which can cause difficulties for my carers. I'll think of three things that need doing and I'll say them instantly before I forget them. That can sound as if I'm hassling, but I'm not actually trying to hurry my carers. Nor am I expecting them to do all three things at once. I'm just giving them advance warning. But it can really throw them. And it's made worse if they happen to be visual people. I have an exceptionally good verbal memory, but, although I respond very well to the visual world, I have no visual memory. Visual people can have real trouble with all my verbal instructions, especially if I give them three at once. I asked someone once to pull me; she pushed me. I felt like asking, as Shakespeare's Parolles was asked, 'Is it a language I speak?' In a sense, we do speak different languages.

I also tend to ask for something to be done when I see that it needs to be done, but I don't expect carers to interrupt what they are doing. What I really mean is: 'When it's convenient, please will you do such and such'. After they've been coming to me for a while, they understand. The worst part of my 24 hours is the time I spend awake in bed; the only time I'm comfortable is when I'm asleep. At first, I would sleep reasonably deeply until around 5 o'clock. That was six hours' sleep, give or take, and as my doctor brother-in-law has reassured me that we need less sleep as we get older, I accepted that. Maybe, I'd have liked more but I could cope with that amount. This was when I was getting myself up in the morning and I'd mostly get up around 6 o'clock, not because I was bursting to go to the lavatory but because the longer I lay there, the more spastic I became. Bed, which should be the most comfortable place, was shockingly uncomfortable. Getting up at that time made for a very long day, so I'd try, if I possibly could endure it, to stay in bed by listening to the radio and trying to distract myself from my body's discomfort. As well, I had the curtain cords extended so that I could, if it wasn't too cold, pull the curtains open and look out onto the apricot tree.

But then my world changed and I had to stay in bed until the carer came at 7 o'clock. My hour of misery had extended itself into two hours. But worse was to come: quite recently I have taken to waking after only three hours' sleep. I don't usually start spasming that early. Instead, I have developed a nervous twitch. Discomfort builds up, say in the left groin, until that leg bends vigorously and then, just as vigorously, straightens. It is more often the left leg, although both legs can be affected. I'd then describe it as knitting. Apart from the acute discomfort, there is a great risk of my gouging pieces out of my legs with my toenails and an even greater risk that my legs will cross. This can be most uncomfortable but is also potentially dangerous. I have such poor circulation that a crossed leg is to invite ulcers. This kicking often continues for the rest of the night, that is from 2.30 a.m. until 7 o'clock. One night, in despair, I put on the radio. During the 15 minutes or so of a Bach oboe concerto, the left leg kicked 12 times. On a night like this, I can feel that I haven't been back to sleep at all and, yet, the time has passed somewhat faster than I would have expected. Either, I am snoozing a little between each kick, or I drop off kicking and wake kicking, so the blessed sleep in between passes unnoticed. I may not be manic-depressive like Hopkins but his line haunts me: 'I wake and feel the fell of dark, not day'.

Recently, this sort of night was usual and a relatively good night was a rarity. I was becoming more and more tired, and more and more dispirited. It was no good my lying down during the afternoon. I'd tried it in Chile. I couldn't go to sleep so I just spasmed my way through the rest time, occasionally snoozing, unrestfully. I was becoming increasingly convinced that, after so many years of holding out against anti-spasm, I'd have to give in and take the dreaded pills. Relief came from an unexpected quarter: the vet. It was cat flu injection time once again and a friend bundled the cats into separate boxes, Fox, as ever, protesting vigorously. I don't think he's afraid. I think it's more that he objects to the loss of dignity. There were several signs that he had been bothered by lower backache, so I asked the vet to check him out. He agreed it was probably arthritis and offered me the choice of two pills: one, conventional medicine, the other, which he said he was taking himself for his RSI, a naturopathic one, proflavanol, an antioxidant made from grape seed. I opted for the second one and duly organised for Fox to have a quarter of a tablet twice a day. As he is notoriously difficult to get pills into, we successfully concealed the pill in a teaspoon of tinned food, which he mostly swallowed on the first attempt.

Almost immediately, I noticed improvements. He started moving more freely, without the stiff-legged gait one associates with an older cat. He is, after all, 13 years old. He had loosened up considerably, *and* he was less grumpy. I had wrongly assumed that the grumpiness was a function of his age and his naturally cussed temperament. I, even, sometimes used to laugh at him. I was wrong and I feel quite ashamed. He must have been in pain. After the first trial fortnight, I rang the vet to confirm I'd be keeping Fox on the pills. He insisted that I might also benefit from the proflavanol and, in the end, persuaded me to give it a month's trial. I had been having a lot of neck, shoulder and left arm pain and I thought, if it was helping the vet's RSI, it might well help that. It had no effect at all on the pain, but it greatly improved the quality of my sleeping pattern. In the first 14 or so days after I started taking Fox's pills, I had three excellent nights of sleep, half a dozen very good nights and the rest were good, except for one that was very fair. None of them was as bad as the really horrible ones I was having before I started taking the proflavanol. It has been suggested that it could be the St John's wort pills I also take that may have been doing me good. I try those because they are used against neuralgia and sciatica. I don't know for certain; all I can say is that Fox improved and he was not taking St John's wort. It may be that I will have to experiment at some stage, although I am very loath to return to my disturbed nights. It could, even, be the combination of the two. In the meantime, sleep is much more bearable.

Chapter 14

At one stage, just after I'd come out of remission, I had a neighbour who'd had a partial mastectomy and a radium implant. As it was, apparently, a very aggressive cancer and she was pre-menopausal, she fully believed, wrongly as it turned out, that she had been given a death sentence. She was very upfront and we used to talk about the differences in our situations: how she had to learn to die with dignity and grace, whereas I had to learn to live that way. As a result of our conversations, I wrote a poem called 'Life Sentence', the third part of which said exactly what I wanted it to say.

> like the dog chained
> to the chariot wheel
> I have no choice –
> it makes no difference
> whether I'm dragged
> claws screaming and scraping
> or whether I trot docilely –
> I travel the same distance –
> the trick is to consent
> to act as if I have chosen
> this particular journey –
> therein lies the transformation
> of my inner landscape –
> falling precipitous cliffs
> become smiling meadows –
> claustrophobic sycamores
> no longer invade my space
> but shelter gently
> a skirmish of sparrows

I had been proud that I had consented, that I had managed to transform my spiritual landscape. But, now, in my greatly changed circumstances, I have discovered I am once more being 'dragged/ claws screaming and scraping'. I am far from consenting. Sadly, I have had to come to realise that it isn't going to be possible to consent once and for all. I am going to have to work at consenting with each new major deterioration. My needing attendant carers was one such deterioration. Needing to be catheterised will, probably, be the next. Indeed, as I become more and more disabled, the consenting may well become a daily necessity.

So, for now, I have to set to work on myself yet again. Once more, I have to change my attitude. And, perversely, with so many people coming into the house and the draining of my energy that this entails, it has been harder to find the much needed tranquillity and solitude for my inner work. Although I am left on my own at different stages throughout the day, I no longer have the uninterrupted solitude that nourished my creativity and inner quiet. After an hour or so of care and company, I can't just press a switch and return to a state of quietness the moment I am left on my own. I feel frazzled and am left with a lot of new material to process. It is often only in the evenings, when I have three to four hours unattended, that I can feel the peace of the house settle around me.

Over the years, when I have been vulnerable and needy, I have reread favourite books. It seems I haven't had the energy to read anything new. I have found safety and comfort in the nostalgia generated by revisiting old friends. It has become my security blanket. This time, when I first had to deal with my greatly changed circumstances, instead of rereading, I watched, over and over again, the video I had been lent of *Pride and Prejudice*. I got to the stage where I knew large chunks of it by heart. I already knew it well because I had had to teach it so often, but this endless rewatching was ridiculous. In the end, I took it as a barometer of how much I was struggling, and rather than castigating myself for my obsession, I laughed gently. I comforted myself with Hopkins's 'My own heart let me more have pity on'. Eventually, I broke myself of this obsession and even took the step of having the television moved into the big room. As I sit in there only in the evenings, and not every evening at that, I cannot often get into a mindless state of doing nothing but watch videos.

Instead, I spend as many hours as I can out in the garden or here in my sitting room looking out the window at the little sky I can see between the branches of my walnut tree and at the sparrows and waxeyes at the bird feeders. But even my time in the garden has changed. I was one who the doctor described as 'fiercely independent'. Yet, now, wherever I am, I stay until someone comes to move me. And the less I do for myself, the less I can do. So, if I am put outside on my wheelchair with my feet on my stool and I get either too hot or too cold, or it begins to rain, once I have taken my feet off the stool, I have no guarantee I'll be able to get them back up again. Sitting with my feet down for any length of time is not a good idea. I have such poor circulation that blood pools in my feet. Even with them up nearly all day, they are permanently, slightly swollen with oedema. As I can't change my position in the garden, I can't go and watch the fish in their barrel or observe the canaries in their aviary or count how many daffodils have come up under my walnut tree – my gardener has just planted 100 – so my time is less varied. Sometimes, my feet spasm off the stool and, with great difficulty, I can manage to put them back; if I am successful, it takes me up to 10 minutes. I just have to calculate when the carer will turn up so that, 20-30 minutes before, I can risk having the feet down long enough for me to inspect the garden. It's harder to have to stay in one spot in the summer; if I'm in the shade I can get too cold but it's too hot for me to be in the unprotected sun.

> I always knew it would be dire
> but it seemed a long way off no need
> to worry yet I was wrong suddenly
> almost overnight everything
> has changed the future has become the present
> and what I dreaded no longer
> lives at a distance but has moved in –
> it's there beside me as I wake
> each morning when I go out
> it is waiting for my return –
> my world isn't mine any more –
> as if the familiar greens of my garden
> had been tainted to everyone else
> they look the same only I can see
> they're now and for ever a sludge
> of colour menacing and unwelcome –

they say you can get used to anything
but what I want isn't that easy –
I want to transform that menace
that lack of welcome into a state
of grace I want to kiss the beast
and receive with joy the prince –
I want to allow the clammy
shivering frog its chance to display
its hidden heroism I want
to live not this drab reality
but inside a fairy tale
where everything is possible –
I would have liked a happy ending

My life has changed so much inwardly that it feels as if there surely must be visible outward signs. I worry still that I will be diminished by the inexorable degeneration and the accompanying narrowing of my life and its choices. Shortly after I was told the true nature of my illness, my doctor recounted a sad little story that a colleague had told him. This man had been visiting a hospital where he had encountered a woman patient so damaged that she needed to be fed. He had known her in her youth when she was hale and hearty.

'It's dreadful seeing you like this,' he told her.

'Yes, it would be, if it were me,' she countered.

When I heard this, I was in remission and I vowed that, no matter how bad I ultimately became, I would still be me. I had no difficulty with that while my symptoms were still at bay, or even while I was still maintaining my bloody-minded independence, but how about now, when most weeks I leave my property only on a Tuesday evening to go to choir? Most unfortunately, the head of the department where I worked at the university, while acknowledging I was one of their best tutors, dumped me. The department had just passed a resolution that only post-graduate students were to be tutors. My post-graduate studies are well behind me, and even though I asked, with heavy irony, which course he would recommend I enrol for, the head didn't take me up on that point. I couldn't have lost the tutoring at a worse time. I like students, enjoy teaching and the university, for goodness sake, paid me to read. My self-esteem, the person I was, was very bound up with my

work. Without it, I was in danger of losing myself. But fortunately, I'd
had to deal with this issue before.

Many years ago, my doctor was away for several months and he asked
his replacement, the daughter of a friend of mine, as it happened, to
check up on me. It was just after Paul's death and my duodenal ulcer
fiasco. I must have indicated that I felt I was handling a difficult situation
rather well. She looked puzzled, as if she didn't agree that the situation
was indeed difficult. She also claimed that, because I was so housebound
and disabled, I would have lost status. At the time, I felt that remark
said more about her than it did about me. Her comment obviously
stayed in my mind, though, and several years later, I wrote the following
poem, called 'No Less'.

> a grey mid-winter afternoon –
> a ripple of wind in the cabbage tree
> no bird song
> a sleeping circle of cat –
> it is a far cry
> from a rainbow over a coral reef
> from the evening ballroom of St Mark's Square
> from a kangaroo at sunrise –
> but I am no less
> because my world contains only
> a tremor of wind against the greyness
> and the cat silently breathing

If, when I wrote this poem, I could feel so certain that I was not
diminished, then surely I will be able to feel equally certain in the future,
no matter what is in store for me. Certainly, some years ago, another
MS sufferer rang me expressing interest in my yoga class. We talked for
a while. As she was hanging up, she said, 'How good it is to talk to
someone who is a person first and has MS second.' I don't know who
she had been meeting, because all the MS sufferers I knew were people.
Maybe, she'd just been unfortunate.

In remaining myself, I am immensely lucky in that I do not
experience some of the MS symptoms my carers have told me that others
suffer from. I have no cognitive problems or short-term memory loss;
my speech is not slurred nor do I have double vision. Nor, as I have

already mentioned, do I suffer from the excessive tiredness that bothers so many MS sufferers. I attribute that to the constant work I do on my energy levels through yoga and meditation.

I am also lucky in other respects. If I think of the loss experienced by Jacqueline du Pré, when she could no longer play the cello, I am very aware of just how fortunate I am. I have four different activities that have been, and are still, very important to me. I started playing the piano when I was eight – indeed, I caused all sorts of family kerfuffles before I was able to play and in the end Dad had to give up smoking to pay for the lessons – but although I can no longer play, I can still listen, and, by singing in a choir, I still make music with other people. I used to love sitting on a beach looking at the sea and the sky or on the hills looking at them against the sky. Now, I sit in my garden and look at the trees and the sky. My yoga practice is now severely curtailed but I still do regular yoga, an hour a day. The carers have had to learn how to help me.

Music, the natural world, yoga: all essential to my well-being. But the most important aspect of my life is not affected by my condition, other than that I now type with one finger. And that sounds worse than it is because I never did type with more than four. Thinking, talking, teaching, reading, writing are unimpaired. My intellectual life is as rich and healthy as ever.

It is most uncomfortable having an illness that other people find threatening. One Sunday several years ago I had spent the day in a drear solitude. I couldn't seem to get out of my own way. During the afternoon, two friends rang. Quite deliberately, I allowed myself to sound the way I felt, instead of assuming a cheerful voice. Both callers asked me anxiously, what was wrong.

'I've got MS,' I replied.

Whereupon, each of them proceeded to tell me why they'd rung. Neither said, 'That must be rough' or asked, 'Are you having a bad day?' It was as if I hadn't spoken.

There had been a time earlier, shortly after my coming out of remission and Paul's death, when I was being driven to my yoga class by one of my pupils. She'd been in the class for several years but was not a close friend.

I heard myself say to her, 'I live without hope, and with nothing to look forward to.'

It was true then, but I shouldn't have dumped something so heavy on her. If I'd realised what I was going to say, I wouldn't have spoken. She couldn't cope. 'Did you know Sharon's got flu?' she asked me.

Another day, several years later I, this time quite deliberately, said to a friend that my walk was getting worse, I was having trouble getting on and off the exercycle, and was finding it more difficult to play the piano. He also changed the subject. 'Do you remember when so and so came to visit?' he asked.

This time, I retaliated. 'Don't change the subject,' I snapped back.

This led to a bit of a spat but we sorted it out and I'll give him the credit for, on this occasion, responding more sensitively to my needs.

This was not the case another time. He had rung because he wanted to offload some personal problem of his own. I admitted that I was having such a bad day that I had no energy to spare. He asked what was going wrong. I explained that it had taken me 10 minutes to put on my socks and a further five to put on my watch.

He made sympathetic noises, but the next time he rang, he made no reference to these difficulties, didn't ask whether things were better. They had disappeared; he just didn't see them as part of an ongoing problem, and, therefore, likely to recur.

I had similar bothers once when my doctor visited to check on my ears, which were stubbornly resisting the nurse's syringe. He talked brightly for several minutes. After all, I hadn't seen him for well over a year. For someone who is chronically ill, I am astonishingly well. In the end, I pointed out that he hadn't asked how I, or rather how the MS, was.

He looked sheepish. 'Let's replay this,' he said. 'How are you?'

So I told him some of the difficulties I was facing. Now, I know doctors don't deal with such practical issues, but he never again referred to what I'd told him. What I'd said made no impression on him at all.

Again, more recently, I was trying to tell a friend on the phone about how isolated I have been feeling. After I'd told him, he gave me a further minute of his time, before indicating he had to get back to work. Although I can't expect the world to stop because I am feeling poorly, which would be to deny the reality of other people's lives and preoccupations, I felt dismissed.

Last year, one of my students, a married woman in her late 20s, asked me an astonishing question. 'Do you find,' she enquired earnestly, 'that you have to be nicer because you're in a wheelchair?'

'No!' I replied. 'Being in a wheelchair frees me to be more eccentric.'
That is true. I have always been somewhat non-conformist. Now,
people accept my non-conformity more readily. They humour me. I
can hear them thinking, 'Poor dear! She's in a wheelchair, so we must
make allowances for her.'

At my age women become invisible. I suppose that's one of the black
humour benefits of being in a wheelchair: I am decidedly conspicuous.
When I first acquired the scooter, one of my friends wanted me to buy
a witch's hat. And certainly, I dress vividly. I've never been part of the
wallpaper and I don't see any reason why I should start now. The wheelchair draws attention to me, no matter what.

I may seem to be labouring the point but the fact of the matter is
that the MS, which is enormously important to me because I have to
live with it day after day, is only of secondary importance to other people.
They are busy with their own lives. There is even wry humour to be
derived from this situation. I am asked how I am and I reply, 'Oh yes!'
or 'It's a nice day' or 'I'm sitting in the garden' and no one notices that
I haven't really answered.

When I had just come out of remission, I was warned by somebody
from the Multiple Sclerosis Society that I would lose friends. I wouldn't
say that, and I have even made friends since I was wheelchair-bound,
but I think the quality of some of the friendships has changed. In many
cases, it has deepened, but in some, it feels more shallow. But then I
remember our friend, Philip, who developed leukaemia when we were
in London. He came to tell me and, I realise now, I failed him. Because
I didn't want him to die, I couldn't't/wouldn't face the fact that he was
dying. I would like to be able to live that time again, so that I could be
really there for him in his lonely dying. It seems likely that, in the same
way, friends don't want me to be getting worse. They don't articulate to
themselves what they are doing but, as I did with Philip, they are denying
the reality of life for me.

Chapter 15

I have recently encountered a medical model that claims MS sufferers undergo a personality change that makes them, considering the severity of the condition, inappropriately positive and cheerful. Apart from the fact that I know of one person afflicted with MS who spends each day in a state of anger and hostility towards the world, this model is too categorical. I checked it out with my doctor – I have now changed to a young woman doctor – and she, who had never before encountered such a theory, regarded it as simplistic. As for me, I feel it is too generalised. Because of the complexity of the nervous system, MS is a very variable condition. People suffer a great range of symptoms. In my first attack, I had almost totally lost the use of my hands and couldn't play the piano. Despite further attacks, it was to be another 28 years before I had to give up the piano for good, and that was as much to do with loss of balance as anything else. Saying that everyone becomes excessively cheerful is equivalent to saying that everyone gets slurred speech or double vision. This is palpably untrue.

A general theory of this kind denies people's individuality. It ignores the personal in favour of statistical possibility. Maybe it is likely that my speech will be slurred, but, as it happens, I speak very clearly. Maybe it is likely that I will be unnaturally cheerful but my cheerfulness is deliberately adopted; in T. S. Eliot's choice phrase, 'there will be time/ To prepare a face to meet the faces that you meet.' And I have found that when you put on a cheerful mask even if inside you're rotten with grief, after a while, you don't just convince others, you convince yourself. It becomes a self-fulfilling prophecy.

I have encountered, as well, various strange responses to the fact of MS. What is known medically is that I will have had a predisposition and that it is a virus, possibly a very common virus like measles, that has mutated. I have heard, however, a claim that it could have been caused by the glandular fever I had some 18 months before the onset. Jacqueline du Pré, as I understand from a biography, also had glandular fever before her illness began. My local MS society refers to multiple sclerosis as the Viking gene and two of my four grandparents came from Yorkshire. But, undoubtedly, no one knows for sure what causes it or how to treat it. That leaves a lot of leeway for the superstitious or the uninformed to put forward their favourite theories.

I've been a sitting duck for those who believe in reincarnation. Either I've chosen to be ill because of what the experience will teach me – I should be so stupid – or my illness is a result of something unspeakable I've done in a previous life. A friend, knowing my opinion of such a worldview, has twitted me about the brazenness of my sitting here totally unembarrassed by such a conspicuous stigma.

Then there was the woman who said succinctly, 'God only tests you to the limits of your strength'. If one considers trouble spots around the world, this is obviously false. I suppose she was merely intending to express sympathy, but I found her remark far from comforting. In the first place, I hadn't been blaming God and, in the second, I wasn't yet at the limits of my strength, so what else was in store for me?

Another explanation of my illness I initially swallowed whole. I told the Jungian analyst I knew slightly in Melbourne that I had MS.

'Fear,' he announced categorically.

I was in remission at the time and only too willing to believe that something I was doing right was keeping me healthy. Even if it was fear that had brought on my illness in the beginning, obviously, I was dealing with it and would be able to continue to do so. It was my guarantee of permanent good health.

It was only later that my natural scepticism reasserted itself. If my dreams were analysed after I had known that I had a chronic and degenerative illness, it would hardly be surprising if they revealed an element of fear. Only a fool would be unafraid in such circumstances. And how many people had he analysed both before and after they had been diagnosed so that he could know for certain that fear was a necessary component because it had shown up before the onset of the illness? I felt uncomfortable that I had so readily accepted his pronouncement.

On the other hand, there are those people who tell me they're sure that they wouldn't be able to cope as well as I do. But the illness is progressive; it is not a case of coping with it all at once. We don't know what we can cope with until the occasion arises. If I could have seen, at the very beginning of the illness, what I would eventually become, I'm sure I would have said the very same. I'm helped by the fact that I have a stubborn nature, that I possess staying power. If a movement doesn't work the first time, I try again and again until it does. I don't give up easily. I was written this script right from birth. My grandmother took one look at me in my bassinet and said, 'Look at that determined little chin.'

It's also true that I don't fully remember what it was like to walk; I remember, emotionally, the feeling of walking the sheep tracks between Purau and Camp Bay with the wind in my hair, but I don't remember the physical sensation. It's not as if one day I was okay and the next day I was in a wheelchair. I didn't have the horror of an accident that left me paraplegic. It's over five years since I was walking, and that was only a little; I'd lurch myself, using a shower stool as a walking frame, from the bed to the bathroom and back around 4.30 in the morning. I was upright and travelling from A to B, which, I suppose, is a definition of walking.

And I tend to compare the nastiness of now with how it was last year, rather than with how it was before the MS encroached on my life. And I've only once retained a dream where I've been walking freely and that was the merest snippet. Since the MS rampaged, I remember far fewer dreams than I used to, but every so often there's a snatch. If I'm walking, I'm always struggling: waving my arms around in a frantic effort to balance, lurching along wishing I'd brought my elbow crutches, or wondering desperately if I'll make it to the desired spot. Sometimes in Melbourne, when I was still in remission, I'd dream I was stumbling, walking very clumsily. The Jungian analyst always interpreted such dreams as showing that I was psychologically off balance. I wonder what he'd make of my more recent dreams: obviously, I'm falling apart, ontologically insecure. I had decided my Melbourne dreams were my body's response to my condition; after all, I'd always notice an increased precariousness when it was very hot. But I can't make a consistent theory that squares with my present dreams.

Inevitably, as the illness worsens and you have to surrender control over so many aspects of your life, you lose your own power. While I was still moderately independent, I had an interesting conversation with various people from Burwood Hospital, who were interviewing me to see if I were a suitable candidate for a voice recognition programme. They asked me who my neurologist was. I explained I hadn't seen one for over 12 years and that then he'd only told me what I already knew. Who was my doctor? I revealed how little contact I had with him and said I felt that, anyway, he didn't have much interest in MS. Well then, what medication did I take? Vitamin C was my reply.

They were much intrigued. 'It would seem,' they declared, 'that you have retained your own power.'

At that stage, I could agree with them. I don't know to what extent they'd now feel that this is the case, given all the carers I have to accommodate. Mostly, I tell them politely/ask them to do things for me, but the truth of it is that I can do very little for or by myself. I tell a carer what I want to eat and the carer gets it. Is this power? Certainly, it's dependence.

I live in my own house, handle my own finances, am consulted at every stage – in fact, I was forced one day to complain to the occupational therapist and one of the carers that they were talking about me in my presence as if I wasn't in the room, just as people do with children – but would you call this control? My care-giving agency can pull the plug on me at any time on no more pretext than that they cannot provide sufficient carers to meet my needs. If I burnt myself severely again, I know I'd be less likely to get my own way when I said I didn't want to go into hospital. I know I'll feel more in control, more as if I have retained my power when I get my own funding. Then, it will be up to me who I employ. Their loyalty will be for me. I expect that then I will feel less dependent. I will be the one setting the job description to meet my needs. I may still be a prisoner in my own house but I will be the one who has selected and trained the guards.

By the way, the Burwood contingent did decide that I needed a voice recognition programme. Training was set in place but did not go very well. At first it was suggested that the computer could not cope with my extensive vocabulary. But I described someone as 'pusillanimous and patronising' without a hitch. The next notion was that my sentences were too complicated. Right, I thought, I'll give it something basic to digest.

'Bother!' I said clearly, 'it's going to be hot again tomorrow.'

It scrambled every single word. I next tried a line from *Macbeth*: 'Stay not upon the order of your going, but go at once.'

It got only two words wrong. I've, therefore, come to the conclusion that I will have to speak to my computer only in Elizabethan English.

Another programme was tried. This was certainly more accurate; the problem was that you have to pause after every word and my creativity (oops!) doesn't function like that. If you see what I mean.

I know that one day I may have to persevere with it and, certainly, typing this epic with one finger has given me considerable neck ache. And you have to remember that I am changing the position of my legs every five minutes, otherwise they spasm off the stool. That means sliding the computer off my knee and removing the cushion it is resting on. Next I have to rearrange my legs, replace the cushion and half slide/half lift my laptop computer back into place. It's a right rigmarole but, in the meantime, I'm carrying on with my one-finger efforts. E-mail means, at least, that I can send short messages often instead of worrying about longer letters.

I have written this, more than 40,000 words, with one finger in just over a month. It has flowed out of me so fast, I can only conclude that I needed to tell my story. I am haunted by Hopkins's lament: 'what word/ Wisest my heart breeds dark heaven's baffling ban/ Bars or hell's spell thwarts. This to hoard unheard,/ Heard unheeded, leaves me a lonely began'. I had been hoarding this unheard. I am hoping that people will remember some of what I have said, like the friend who re-membered from a line of my poetry that said I was wearing 'a wet suit lined with sandpaper'.

I have come to the end but it is not a very satisfactory end. There is no closure. I am loath to declare it finished once and for all, not just because I may remember something else I want to include, but because my circumstances are changing every day, so there is no ending. As well, autobiographical accounts are notoriously difficult to sustain; they tend to peter out as they come to their final pages. The author is too close to events, too involved. There is no room for the necessary aesthetic distance.

But, for now, I'm here, living in this house on my own with two cats, three fish, eleven canaries and an army of carers. I'm still a vegetarian who does yoga every day. Judging by my family's longevity – three grand-parents and both parents attained the age of 80 or more – I'm likely to live another 20 years. I don't know how severely disabled I'll be or even whether I'll achieve my goal and live in this house until I die. So, I have to leave you hanging. This is how it is for me on a cold winter evening in the big room, with the gas fire humming and two companionably sleeping cats. I'm waiting to be put to bed.

As for tomorrow, I cannot say.